Nervous Disorders of Women

Born in Vienna in 1864, Bernard Hollander was a London-based psychiatrist in the early twentieth century. He is best known for being one of the main proponents of the interest in phrenology at that time. This title, originally published in 1916, looks at 'the numerous nervous illnesses of women, in which the *mental* factor plays a large part, and which are known as functional disorders, as distinguished from organic diseases'. He looks at the role of psychotherapy as an emerging treatment for these disorders. There is also a companion volume which looks at the *Nervous Disorders of Men*.

Nervous Disorders of Women

The modern psychological conception of their causes, effects and rational treatment

Bernard Hollander

Routledge
Taylor & Francis Group
LONDON AND NEW YORK

First published in 1916
by Kegan Paul, Trench, Trubner & Co. Ltd

This edition first published in 2015 by Routledge
27 Church Road, Hove BN3 2FA

and by Routledge
711 Third Avenue, New York, NY 10017

Routledge is an imprint of the Taylor & Francis Group, an informa business

ISBN: 978-1-138-81230-7 (hbk)
ISBN: 978-1-315-74888-7 (ebk)

NERVOUS DISORDERS OF WOMEN

THE MODERN PSYCHOLOGICAL CONCEPTION OF THEIR CAUSES, EFFECTS, AND RATIONAL TREATMENT

BY

BERNARD HOLLANDER, M.D.

AUTHOR OF "THE MENTAL FUNCTIONS OF THE BRAIN", "MENTAL SYMPTOMS OF BRAIN DISEASE", "FIRST SIGNS OF INSANITY", "HYPNOTISM AND SUGGESTION", ETC.

SECOND EDITION

LONDON
KEGAN PAUL, TRENCH, TRUBNER & CO., LTD.
NEW YORK: E. P. DUTTON AND CO.
1916

BY THE SAME AUTHOR

NERVOUS DISORDERS OF MEN

THE MODERN PSYCHOLOGICAL CONCEPTION OF THEIR CAUSES, EFFECTS, AND RATIONAL TREATMENT.

ABNORMAL CHILDREN

(NERVOUS, MISCHIEVOUS, PRECOCIOUS, AND BACKWARD)

A Book for Parents, Teachers, and Medical Officers of Schools.

ILLUSTRATED

First Edition . February, 1916
Second Edition . May, 1916

Printed in Great Britain

PREFACE

THIS volume treats of the numerous nervous illnesses of women, in which the *mental* factor plays a large part, and which are known as functional disorders, as distinguished from organic diseases. It is a companion volume to the one on *Nervous Disorders of Men.* Of course, many of the complaints are common to both men and women; but their causation, and to some extent their treatment, is different in the two sexes and justifies the description being given in separate volumes, although a number of paragraphs in the two books must of necessity be similar or identical.

What has been said of men is still more true of women, that up to quite recent years patients suffering from these disorders were not taken seriously, and their treatment was left largely to persons outside the profession, lay practitionors, specialising in one form of treatment: in electricity, massage, physical exercise, diet treatment, or other specific, and the various "mental healers" of "Christian Science,"

"Higher Thought," and other cults. Needless to say that there is no one method in existence which is a "cure-all." Medicinal, hygienic, dietetic, physical and moral measures have all to be employed according to the individuality of the patient and the nature of the complaint, and it is only a qualified physician who can possess the requisite knowledge.

As in men so in women, the mental, or more correctly speaking, the emotional, factor plays a large part in the causation of nervous disorders, and mental causes require mental treatment. There are various methods of applying it, and it is the purpose of this book to show what can be accomplished by them. Hence this book, although not a textbook, may be of interest and some value to the busy practitioner; and, being written in non-technical language, it should appeal also to lay readers desirous of practical and useful information on the subject of nervous disorders of women, their prevention and treatment, especially to those who have the care of nervous patients.

BERNARD HOLLANDER, M.D.

57 WIMPOLE STREET,
LONDON, W.
November, 1915.

CONTENTS

INTRODUCTION

DIFFERENCES IN THE NERVOUS SYSTEM AND MENTAL DISPOSITIONS OF MEN AND WOMEN

As the female body shows anatomical characters which distinguish it from that of the male, so does the nervous system.

Taking the brain first, as the great centre—the centre of centres—of the nervous system, we notice at once that the average female brain is about one inch smaller in circumference and about five ounces lighter in weight than the average male brain. I am speaking of the average and not of specially endowed women. The difference is perceptible in the infant as well as in the adult, in the savage as well as in civilised races. There is no denying the fact, but, as I shall show, we must not draw from it the conclusion that women are mentally inferior to men.

The smaller size of the female brain is a fundamental sexual distinction, and may be accounted for partly by the hypothesis that environment, educational advantages, and habits of life, acting through a long series of generations, have stimulated the growth of the brain in one sex more than in the other. At the same time we must not forget that the female child inherits as much from the father as from the mother; indeed, boys more often take after their mother and girls after their father.

Some investigators attribute the difference in the weight of the brain to the difference in the bulk of the body. It is true that the general physique of women is less robust than that of men, and that their stature is less. The expectation that a smaller brain would be required might therefore seem reasonable. But we know that there is no such correspondence between the size of the brain and that of the body. Little men often have large brains, and giants small ones.

Whatever may be the explanation of the undoubted fact that the average woman's brain is smaller than that of the average man, we do not share the opinion of those scientists—and there are many of them—who deduce from this fact the argument that women are less intellectual than men. Very few brains of women of distinction have been examined by the anatomist; and the women dying in hospitals, whose brains do come under inspection, are of an inferior type. Moreover, there have been eminent men with very small and abnormally light brains. It is obvious, therefore, that no inference can be drawn from such observations as to the relation between the size and weight of the brain and the intellectual capacity of the individual.

The late Professor Bischoff, of Munich, one of the chief physiologists of Europe, asserted the mental inferiority of women against men, basing his opinion chiefly on the fact which he claimed to have observed, that the average weight of a man's brain is $49\frac{1}{2}$ ounces, but a woman's only 44 ounces. After his death, the post-mortem examination revealed that his own brain weighed only $43\frac{7}{8}$ ounces, i.e. slightly less than his own estimate of the average weight of women's brains.

There is another valid reason against the assumption of inferiority of intellect because of the smaller brain-size and weight, and that is that the brain has many functions to perform. The intellectual operations are only one of them; therefore the size of the entire brain gives no clue whatever as to the intellectual capacity of man or woman. If it did, what about animal brains? Some animals, even after all allowance has been made for the size of the body, have larger brains than man, and yet none of them approach even the lowest type of man in intellect.

The fact is that the size of the entire brain is not a measure of intellectual capacity at all. It is a measure of capacity of all the energies taken together, that is of the animal instincts and passions, the feelings as well as the intellect. The intellectual region, as we now know, is confined to the frontal lobes, the most anterior part of the brain. A man or woman may have a large head and yet be stupid, if the frontal region be small; and he or she may have a small head with great wisdom, if the greater mass of brain be in the anterior region.

Most investigators have hitherto disregarded this distinction, and treated the brain as if it had only one function—the manifestation of intellect. Consequently they argued that, since the brain of woman weighs about five ounces less than that of man, therefore, on merely anatomical grounds, we might expect a marked inferiority of intellectual power in the female sex. Whereas it is now shown that this difference in brain-weight does not explain whether the deficiency lies in intellect, in strength of sentiment, or force of brute propensity.

It is evident that the intellectual functions must be related to a part of the brain which, as regards its size, distinguishes the human brain from that of animals, and this is the case as regards the frontal lobes. In animals we find only rudiments of frontal lobes corresponding to their comparative weakness of reasoning power; and there is a difference in their size in man in accordance with the intellectual capacity of different races. That the frontal lobes alone are concerned with the higher intellectual operations has been demonstrated by experimental investigation, as well as by the observation of the effects of injury and disease on the human brain. Moreover, careful measurements have shown that education tends to increase the volume of the anterior part of the brain.

What we want, therefore, is a comparison of the size and weight of the frontal lobes of men and women, educated and uneducated. The only measurements in existence were taken many years ago, and do not include cultured women. Therefore, though we have on record weights and measurements of brains of women of the uneducated classes, further evidence is necessary before we can draw any satisfactory conclusions. There can be no doubt that when women cultivate their intellect, the frontal lobes of the brain do grow.

Women's brains are narrower than men's, they are smaller in the so-called motor area, and in the part which we have in common with animals; therefore they exhibit less force, less energy, and less animal passion altogether.

On the other hand, quite a number of observers, such as Huschke, Broca, Crichton-Browne and others, have noted that the posterior part of the brain is more voluminous in women than in men; in other words, that women are more long-headed, and this part, according to some old theories, confirmed by quite recent investigators, appears to be concerned with the manifestation of the feelings and emotions which we know to be stronger in women.

This posterior area (the somatic sensory area of Flechsig) is related by means of the sympathetic nervous system with the organs of the chest and abdomen, from which sensations which have to do with our unconscious vegetative life are conveyed to the brain. We know that, when the emotions are very active, they influence the functions of the bodily organs according to the mental state of the person; thus it is that we feel our emotions have their seat, not in our heads but in our bodies. The languages of all nations refer the emotions to the heart, in and about which organ are grouped large masses of the great sympathetic system.

This sympathetic or ganglionic nervous system, which is not under our voluntary dominion, must be distinguished from the cerebro-spinal nervous system which supplies all the muscles and organs over which—in the normal state—we have more or less voluntary control. It consists, in the first place, of a double chain of ganglia, over fifty in number, extending from the base of the brain along the sides of the whole spinal column; in the second place, of certain ganglia scattered among the thoracic, abdominal, and pelvic viscera; and in the third place, of an almost infinite number of nerve-cords distributed over the entire body. These sympathetic nerve-cords supply, firstly, the voluntary or cerebro-spinal nervous system, thus exerting a control over our intentional movements; secondly, the coats of all the arteries controlling the local blood-supply and thus nutrition; and, thirdly, all organs of the interior of the body are supplied more or less abundantly with sympathetic nerves.

Sufficient notice has not been taken of the fact that in women the sympathetic or ganglionic nervous system, which controls the vegetative and sensitive life, is more developed than in man, one reason being that it has to supply some additional organs not existing in man, the breasts, the womb, and the ovaries. Women having more organs concealed in the pelvis than men, and with a greater number of functions to perform, their sympathetic nerves are more numerous. It is due in part to this more elaborate sympathetic system that women feel more keenly the emotional side of mental life. Their affections are deeper, they are more subject to fear, shock, and fright, more readily roused to joy and sorrow, and their grief is more intense. It is through the sympathetic nervous system that tears are shed in grief, that the salivary and gastric secretions are checked in terror, that the milk-flow is increased, arrested or altered under the influence of maternal love, terror, and rage, and that the peristaltic action of the bowels is influenced by certain strong emotions, such as sudden fear. It is owing to the influence of the sympathetic system over the calibre of the blood-vessels that women blush more readily, and blushing is most frequent at the time when the pelvic organs assume their functions, i.e. at puberty.

The ancients referred hysteria, a nervous and mental disturbance peculiar to women, to the pelvic organs, and there is no doubt a connection. Not that the disease is seated there, but these organs form part of a reflex arc to the brain-centres by means of the sympathetic system, which in hysteria is probably in a state of hyperæsthesia. The reason why modern women are less subject to hysteria than their great-grandmothers were, is because of their reason and self-control being trained at the expense of their emotional nature, and because of the modern outdoor life and greater activity in general strengthening the voluntary or cerebro-spinal nervous system, which in many respects acts as a check to the sympathetic.

We have seen, then, that judging by her brain and nervous organisation, woman is mentally not inferior to man, she is only dissimilar. The preponderance of the emotional nature in woman would incline her to seek happiness in the gratification of her feelings rather than her intellect; hence though a woman may be intellectually equal to man, she has not the motive to exert her thinking faculties to the same extent as man has, even though she have the gift and energy to persevere. We all require a motive to work, and we are all happy only to the extent to which we can gratify our natural dispositions. Man knows he will have to earn his living, not only to keep himself, but his wife and family; he must provide for their future; so he is put in early years to hard manual or intellectual labour, and if his parents have no or but modest means, he is aware that the knowledge he acquires will be his only capital. His emotions are not so strong as woman's and are more readily kept in check by the intellect. On the other hand, woman, however gifted she be by nature, has rarely the same strength of impulse to exert her powers to the utmost. If she had, there is no reason why she should not equal man, or even excel him, as is evident from the brilliant way in which many women have acquitted themselves at examinations.

We need only look at the heads of women to see that their frontal brain is not inferior to that of men, and that consequently there is as much material for intellectual training as there is in men. At the same time it is a fact that the ordinary woman is more under the influence of the feelings, that she looks at things differently, and is prompted by different motives to the use of her energies. Modern training may alter this; in any case, I hope to have proved that there is no question of superiority or inferiority of one sex as compared with the other.

If man's intellect is frequently superior, both as to originality and the capacity for amassing knowledge, woman has a greater refinement of nervous organisation, which gives her a rapidity of perception and a rapidity of thought which appear as intuitive insight. Man's mind is as a rule more deductive, woman's more intuitive. In man reflective analysis predominates, in woman spontaneous synthesis. A woman often judges single cases rather than principles ; she is better fitted for forming particular ideas than for generalisation and abstraction. Man may appear to have better judgment, woman frequently has more sagacity. Her thinking is more feeling, and she is strongest when impelled by emotion.

Much has been made of the fact that women have shown little creative and inventive power, that even in such occupations as tailoring, hairdressing, and cooking men seem to excel, and that even domestic appliances and the machinery for knitting, spinning, weaving, and sewing have been invented by men, although there is no reason why women should not have exercised their minds on these improvements. It is also frequently pointed out that music is one of those arts which were always open to women. In it she could express all the emotions of her nature. Yet how many great women composers are there? This absence of inventive and artistic genius may be to some extent accounted for, firstly, by the fact that women do not come so much in contact with other minds as men do, or used not to, and do not receive the same amount of stimulus; and secondly, by their emotional and domestic life taking up too much of their time and energy. Man has said for ages that the "helpmeet for him" shall do the drudgery of looking after him, or at any rate of seeing that it is done; he has dubbed himself the lord of creation, and has consistently paraded the subjugation of his partner. On occasions he has found it convenient to delegate some of his functions to his hitherto submissive partner, and he is now beginning to be rather rudely awakened to the fact that the partner has equal rights.

Man can devote himself entirely to his intellectual work; even in love and in marriage it is only after his daily task is completed that he need give vent to his emotions. He has not the same domestic responsibilities and can thus concentrate his energies and attention on his work. Man gets stimulated by his outdoor life, coming in contact with other minds; woman, living at home, meets only a few intimates and has her intellectual sphere soon narrowed down to the small events of the household. It is due to this difference in the sphere in which they move that men's sufferings arise chiefly from exhaustion, those of women from restricted energies. This is shown so often in times of trouble when no amount of work can make woman ill. It is usually in inactivity that symptoms of illness and disintegration appear in her.

Woman's refined nervous organisation renders her sensibility so keen that she is quick to feel the suffering or joy of others, and to read by the slightest external signs what passes within. Many women will see at a glance whether things have gone well or ill with one, whether one has been pleased or fretted, known failure or success, and especially whether one loves her still. It is this insight and exquisite gift of sympathy which renders woman so invaluable in the chamber where sickness droops and pines. Love for dumb animals, affection for children, commiseration for the weak and helpless, regard for the aged and the suffering, pity for the oppressed—all these are natural to most women.

The failings of men are those of strength, those of women of weakness. The consciousness of the lack of muscular strength has given rise to the petty acts and petty ways which women have had to adopt for securing their aims. Woman's sense of weakness makes her timid; yet the delicate female, who could tremble and turn pale at the very sight of a warlike instrument, or even a mouse, will oftentimes bear the pains of sickness and the approach of death with more serenity and fortitude than the soldier of a hundred battles. The heroism of man is recorded in history; woman's heroism, however, is much commoner, though displayed where there are none to chronicle its victories.

I have already pointed out that girls more often take after their fathers and boys after their mothers, not only in likeness, but in organisation and character. Thus nature prevents extremes of manly and womanly qualities. There are thousands of women with both the brains and the character-qualities of men, just as there are thousands of men who possess the brain-organisation and mental peculiarities of women. It is the training which girls receive which accentuates their female qualities, just as the training which boys receive accentuates their manly characteristics. As long as men are free agents from youth upwards, and women only attain to even comparative freedom when middle-aged, it is clearly impossible to say with certainty whether their apparent shortcomings in the matter of general intelligence are due to natural defects or to environment.

Many generations have cultivated the belief that woman is fundamentally inferior to man; and some of the feminine characteristics, in the exaggerated form at least, are due quite as much to the inherited influence of this concept of woman, which she was trained to share, as to a natural difference in sex. Woman's effort at self-emancipation, however misdirected and attended with absurdities, is, primarily, instinctive resistance to her declared natural inferiority to man, and to the restriction of her capacities it imposes. The woman movement was not caused because there are fewer men inclined to marry, but, primarily, by woman's protest against the estimate of her as a woman that was rejected by the deeper instincts of her nature; and, secondarily, by the disappointing, and often repelling, experience of marriage; for the marriages where there has been no disillusion—though all too often on both sides, it is true—are so few as to constitute exceptions to the rule. A smothered sense of injustice, increasing in strength with each generation as education covered wider fields of knowledge, broke forth finally in a "new woman" who, unwisely assertive at times, declared her right to fill, at her own option, any sphere for which she possessed capabilities, instead of being limited to the only one allowed her on the basis of her natural inferiority.

There is more than one species of the "new woman"; all do not ape masculinity, or hold it an ideal to be attained. The truly newest of the "new" values her womanliness too highly to part with it, is as ready to see the limitations of her own as of the other sex, the expediency of not attempting to do that which the other sex can do better; but she claims the right, as one half of the unit, Man, to think and judge for herself; to be as capable of self-direction, and of consequent building of character, as the other half. The "new woman" is not averse to marriage, but objects to what marriage has been made by this idea of inferiority, whose logical consequence is her submission to superiority; an idea that has permitted and encouraged a double standard of morality. Neither above nor below, but side by side and shoulder to shoulder, is the attitude for marriage she defends as wise and necessary; so that both, dissimilar from the beginning, may prepare for their united office by filling first, most worthily, each their distinctive office. While the "new woman" may prefer to have a man provide for her, she does not feel herself incapable, nor does she wish to be considered incapable, of providing for herself. It is the idea of woman as an incapable, to which the "old woman" with inward protest submitted, that the "new woman" with uttered protest resents; while she accepts rationally, as well as sentimentally, her position as "helpmeet," bringing to it a prepared fitness and force of character that will ennoble the position as the position ennobles the woman. Woman's dependence has made her seek to attract man and to gain power over him, by craft if need be ; but woman's awakened self-respect and self-reliance disdains the craft and demands mutual recognition of equality with difference, mutual dependence and support, mutual aim and accomplishment—a nobler manhood and womanhood, better conditions for the coming generations, through the helpfulness of one for the other, of which both are in need.

NERVOUS DISORDERS OF WOMEN

CHAPTER I

CAUSES OF NERVOUS DISORDERS IN WOMEN

"NERVOUSNESS" is the trouble of the age. Many men and women are never really ill, nor well either, that is to say, they are never ill enough to be confined to bed, and never well enough to enjoy either work or pleasure. They may not complain of their "nerves" at all, nor do they always suspect that their nervous system is at fault; but they think that some particular organ is diseased, for which they seek treatment. Some suffer from dyspepsia without any recognisable disease of the stomach; some from cardiac troubles with an apparently sound heart; some from muscular weakness or spinal pain, without suspecting their nervous system to be at fault, and others from altered secretions from organs apparently in a normal state.

There may be no local disturbances, but only general debility and depression, a state in which the patient can do nothing so well as formerly, and finds every little exertion a trouble; and often this is accompanied by a feeling of insecurity and self-distrust, the patient becoming nervous, easily agitated, over-sensitive, emotional, and timid. The ills of these patients are neither imaginary nor invented; and while they do not necessarily confine them to bed, they often prove the source of such serious disturbances as to make them very miserable.

Numerous volumes have been written on this subject of functional disorders of the nervous system, but most of them are the work of persons unqualified to express scientific opinions, charlatans, and exponents of alleged specific cures or of pseudo-religious cults. Yet it is important that the diagnosis of functional disease should be carefully made, for even in chronic organic cases many important changes take place without the accompanying physical signs; and to determine the question whether an ailment is functional or organic will at times mystify even the most competent and skilful physician.

As in other diseases, so in nervous disorders, we must first of all endeavour to ascertain the cause. Often, when it is possible to remove the source of irritation, the patient will recover without any other help. Of course, a cure is not always so easy, for hereditary disposition plays a conspicuous part; and the predisposition of character and temperament thus derived has, in many cases, been aggravated by faults in education and training.

Excessive physical exercise may produce fatigue and nervous exhaustion. But this sort of fatigue does not occur often in women and, if it does, is not dangerous. It must be pushed to an extreme before it gives rise to exhaustion. Ordinary fatigue from physical exercise is not to be feared, because, from inherent laziness, we stop working long before it could possibly be hurtful.

Fatigue caused by intellectual overwork occurs chiefly in girl students. Intellectual work is less hygienic than physical work, for intellectual work demands a sedentary life and a sitting posture. It chills the extremities by bringing the blood to the head. Yet it does little harm when not accompanied by worry.

The fatigue that is most common in women is caused by emotional excess. Such fatigue is harmful in the highest degree. It is impossible for them to avoid emotional fatigue completely. Most women are naturally highly emotional.

Their affections are very strong. They take things to heart easily. They cannot stand emotional shocks for long. Nervous disorders are particularly common in women who have sorrows or experienced disappointments, and have to keep their grief and worries to themselves. However, it is not always real misfortune which disturbs their physical health; it is more often the trifling nothings, the petty annoyances, and the pin-pricks of life in an impressionable, sensitive woman that cause emotional reactions, which by their constant repetition produce nervous exhaustion.

An emotional cause nearly always exists, though it may have disappeared from the patient's field of consciousness. She may be haunted by the memory of something that is no more and can never be again; or the future may cause her anxiety, either her own or that of someone who is very dear to her. These are the situations in which one cannot see any bright outlook. The emotional cause may be in the realm of the affections or in the sexual sphere. Frequently it consists of memories to which the patient cannot get accustomed and which, though repressed, still disturb the patient's mind and nervous system. Sometimes it is a conflict between her reason and her feelings which is the cause of the psycho-neurosis. It is particularly apt to occur in women who have to keep worries to themselves. The normal woman knows how to forget or, at least, how to distract herself; while in those predisposed, the emotion leads to persistent preoccupation. With the same cause very different effects may follow according to the individual predisposition.

An emotion tires the organism, and particularly the nervous system, more than the most intense physical or intellectual work. We all know the effect of terror or anger; but even simple ill-humour caused by those who surround us can take away all our enthusiasm and energy. And let us note the fact that if the conduct of others has been the cause of our emotion, it is really we ourselves who have created it by the manner in which we have reacted. The mischief is in our mode of reaction to emotional stimuli. An excessive reaction is often congenital and aggravated by faulty education. True, we often see women who tell us they enjoyed good health up to a certain date; but if we take the trouble, by frequent conversations, to scrutinise the mental past of those patients and to analyse their previous state of mind, we find no difficulty in recognising that, long before the development of the actual trouble, the nervous tendency was traceable, and the event that brought on the acute symptom was only like the drop of water that made the vessel overflow.

Thousands of women are rendered exceedingly nervous and held in social bondage by their foolish endeavours to shine in society and the desire to be regarded as somebody. On the other hand, the life of the average housewife and mother is also often made one of unnecessary drudgery and useless anxiety. With some the methods of living are extravagant, and this results in producing dissatisfaction and discontent on the part of those who have not the necessary means. Or else it is merely the abnormal " rush " through life which is the cause, due in some instances to an exaggerated idea of their own importance, in others to an overestimation of the importance of the work they are doing. Many of these women bustle about industriously, but they are accomplishing little in the line of real, useful work. These chronically rushed women keep both mind and body working under a terrible strain, until by and by this state of strain becomes habitual and they cannot relax.

Even some of the conspicuous and peculiar virtues of women may, if unguided and undisciplined, become sources of trouble in one inclined to nervousness. Unselfishness may drive her into giving up necessary rest or sleep or diversion; and strong affections or sympathy may lead her into emotional excess, which is one of the most extravagant forms of nervous expenditure. When such emotional excesses have acted long enough and are followed by debilitating influences, like loss of blood, diseases, physical and mental shocks, or most potent of all, by prolonged anxiety and hard bodily work, such as is entailed in nursing someone dear to her, with the usual accompaniment of irregular hours, loss of sleep, and hasty meals at irregular intervals, we have a combination which will almost certainly result in nervous breakdown.

Some women are preoccupied with matters upon which no amount of taking thought can be of the slightest avail, and with regard to questions which are not deserving of the anxiety bestowed upon them. They are born "worriers." Their minds are engrossed with small points that irritate them, or filled with apprehensions of what is about to go wrong. To those on the look-out for something to trouble about there is usually no dearth of material; yet sometimes, it does seem to the onlooker that the subjects on which they seize betray, by their far-fetched character, the fact that life near at hand must be singularly free from real sorrow. Many of these women are hypersensitive. They worry because they think themselves neglected or slighted, or are criticised either justly or unjustly by their best friends. Other good women are dejected because they are sure that their great worth is not fully appreciated. Still others fret and fume and worry because they feel it is their duty to resent some supposed or real injury or injustice which has been done to them.

No wonder such women complain that they cannot remember what they ought to remember, for they cannot forget what ought to be forgotten—the things that are unpleasant, the things that irritate, the things that make them feel bitter and unkind. By forgetting their disappointments, their annoyances, the wrongs that have been done to them, indeed all the disagreeable things, they would develop a sunny disposition, a good-natured temper, a cheerful manner, a healthful body. Forgetting disagreeable things keeps at bay wrinkles and old age. It beautifies the countenance with a beauty all its own, that of peace and contentment. How can they forget ? By turning their minds to happier things, taking up a book to read, or going out into the fresh air, by filling their minds so full of other matters that there will be no room for the unpleasant memories. By learning to forget, the memory has fewer things to remember and will become stronger and more alert as regards the things it ought to remember.

In many women it is simply misdirected energy which is at the root of their nervous disorder. We are educating our women much more highly than used to be the case, yet few ever take advantage of such education. As regards a good many, who get married, the education received is of little use to them, or they do not understand how to make use of it; and the monotony of domestic life, the lack of varied intellectual interests, the continual or exclusive occupation with the small and uninspiring details of household management which characterise the lives led by many women, help the development of nervousness in a different way. A woman bound down to work of this kind, with brain-energy for which she has no outlet, is liable to exaggerate the importance of trifles, is apt to cultivate worries, and to end, at best, in losing her sense of mental and moral perspective, exaggerating small faults of her own or of others. She is likely, too, as happens in anyone excluded from larger interests or wider contact with the world, to permit her own views and personal peculiarities to grow until they reach an undue size and strength and become difficult to control.

It was different with the woman of olden times. She had to manufacture many things which are now obtained ready-made, so that her brain was kept active; she had a number of children, the care of which kept her busy and left her no time for introspection. Whereas now the refinements of modern life, the corrupt air of crowded cities, the change from the active housekeeper of our forefathers' time to the vacuity of mind of the ornamental woman of the present epoch, the alteration from the period when women were happy to have children to the present time when women in every station of life sedulously seek to diminish the number of their offspring—these and many other changes in the life of the women of to-day undoubtedly tend to increase the proportion of nervous disorders.

Women of the leisured class are frequently without any interest that will save them from themselves; they have nothing that they absolutely *must* do. In many cases their nervous ailments are due to nothing more than lack of proper occupation of mind. Many women have nothing serious with which to occupy themselves.

They are not obliged to get up in the morning if they do not want to, or at least any excuse, however slight, serves to keep them in bed. Very often there are either no children or the mother has nothing to do with her children early in the morning. Without any real occupation of mind, the mind occupies itself with the body and emphasises every sensation, evokes new pains and aches, and the consequence is likely to be a highly neurotic state.

Others have interests, but none that create obligations, that arouse a sense of duty, none that absorb them. It is quite impossible that such women should be either happy or healthy. The occupation of a woman, unlike that of a man, holds out little future for her. It does not arouse her ambition. The daily work of those who have to earn their living is often a monotonous grind that must be endured for the sake of the wages that it brings.

Whereas the sufferings of man arise chiefly from exhaustion, those of the woman arise, above all, from restricted energies. Girls brought up for marriage only have their nervous system upset by the uneasy time of waiting. They attend balls which disappoint them, go into company which bores them, take part in family intercourse which leaves them weary. If they remain spinsters, the want of congenial occupation, sometimes loneliness, neglect, disappointment, and anxiety as to the future tend to produce an unhealthy state of mind which is a primary condition for the development of nervous disorders. Therefore sensible women look about them for something which can give their idle days a purpose, the emptiness of their existence a meaning.

Girls must be brought up to have a proper aim in life. For the cultivated woman love is not a compelling force. When the entire bringing-up and education of the girl is directed to one end only—to get her united to the "right" man—it often happens that, as soon as that object is achieved, all the intellectual interests which the girl pursued are neglected; for there never was a strong, natural desire for the studies so affected. Those who have followed their intellectual inclinations seriously as a rule keep up their interests notwithstanding domestic duties.

Marriage frequently is an episode in the life of man, but it nearly always is an epoch in that of woman; hence the problem of happiness or unhappiness of marriage is of much greater consequence to women than to men. Marriage is a lottery, in which men stake their liberty and women their happiness. There are all those marriages in which there is not a spark of enthusiasm on either side, where husband and wife only seek to get along tolerably with one another. Even if we exclude the decidedly unhappy ones, for which separation or divorce is the proper remedy, there are many women whose husbands are not what their heart and head desires, and who suffer mentally if not physically—and perhaps unknown to anyone but themselves. A man gets away from his domestic misery, he has his business to attend to; but a woman is reminded all day long of what is and what might have been. She may conceal her married troubles and exhibit a false appearance of happiness, she may even do her best to deceive herself and gain for herself an outward content; but such repression of her emotions is not good for her.

Then there are those ill-matched marriages of the weaker husband and physically stronger wife or the strong husband and the delicate wife. In both these unfortunate unions, the wife's nervous system is liable to be injured. Attention must be called to the danger young girls, still ignorant of the world, run by marrying men advanced in years. With the great majority of men who have delayed marriage the freshness and cleanness of youth is gone, and their wives have to be content with the worn and soiled manhood that is left. Even if they do not bring actual disease as their marriage gift, and they be free from degraded tastes, there are other circumstances in the relations between such husbands and wives which render the latter liable to become neurotic and ailing.

Amongst young women of a marriageable age there is often a great deal of ignorance concerning reproductive functions, and a still greater amount of half-knowledge, which is more dangerous than either total ignorance or the fullest information. These mistaken methods of secrecy have often the most unfortunate effect of stimulating the imagination. Novels and theatrical plays which appeal to the sensual passion, modern dances and the free access to the daily newspaper which brings into prominence the libidinous details of every divorce case, all these influences excite in the young morbid feelings which after a time upset the nervous equilibrium.

On the other hand, even the healthiest woman has periods when her nervous system and with it her mental state are liable to become temporarily unstable. She has her periodic menstruation, which reacts on her brain and nervous system; she is subject to nutritional disturbances during pregnancy and confinement, which affect her disposition in greater or slighter degree; and lastly, there is the "change of life," which few women undergo without some nervous disturbances.

Finally, anæmia and exhausting diseases cause defective nutrition of the nerve centres, thus diminishing their resistance and rendering them more vulnerable; and all forms of poisoning, whether by auto-intoxication or the drink or drug habit, are apt to produce nervous symptoms.

CHAPTER II

NERVOUS EXHAUSTION. LOSS OF PHYSICAL AND MENTAL ENERGY

ONE of the commonest forms of nervous disorder is nervous exhaustion. The first sign is usually a " tired " feeling without adequate cause. The least exertion, such as a short walk, produces an inordinate sense of fatigue and weariness even in women who to all appearances are in good muscular condition. They can make strong single or brief exertions, but cannot continue to apply their forces. The weakness lies not in the muscles but in the nerve-centres that control them, which are too readily exhausted. The nutrition of these nerve-centres is defective and the fatigue experienced is only a sign of it.

I have seen nervous women who at the consultation let themselves go all to pieces and flop upon the sofa. To see them one would believe that one was looking at a patient in a faint or dying. However, examination reveals that the pulse is strong, regular, and of normal frequency ; the respiration is normal, or a little hurried by reason of anxiety; the skin is normal in colour and the muscles are well developed. The helplessness of the patient is in striking contrast with her bodily appearance.

The patient finds that her legs soon get tired, and by degrees she becomes conscious of the fact that exercise is no longer a source of enjoyment. Lassitude is constant and hinders the commencement of any activity, renders its execution painful, and is so little mitigated by rest that it is by no means uncommon to hear a patient complain that she is as tired after a night's rest as when she went to bed. This tired feeling tends to increase until late in the afternoon, when, curiously enough, she usually begins to improve. Some of these patients find it impossible to make an effort, while others are capable of effort and of considerable physical work, and only complain of subsequent fatigue being too strongly felt. As a rule the fatigue which is due to a diminution of nervous energy not only comes on quickly but is also very lasting.

Any form of activity which involves the co-ordinated use of certain muscles quickly brings on a feeling of fatigue in these muscles. Thus the victim finds that her arms tend to fall limply to her sides after she has kept them for a few minutes in the position assumed in doing up the hair. In others the throat feels easily tired, and the voice becomes husky and broken after a short conversation. Still others find that even the effort involved in writing a few lines causes more or less discomfort, and that this feeling becomes so marked that perseverance is all but impossible; a letter which begins with characters that are firm and legible ends in an illegible and disjointed scrawl. The patient cannot exert herself; friends, household, books, amusements, her usual occupations all fail to do anything except add to her fatigue.

It is not only in the physical domain that these patients are helpless. The consciousness of helplessness extends also to the moral domain, and the trivial ground on which the patient feels discouraged indicates the exaggerated degree of nervous reaction. The memory may become impaired owing to the power of attention being diminished. There may be a difficulty of recalling proper names, dates, and even single words such as the names of articles in daily use. Conversation becomes painful, the patient being unable to preserve the thread of her thoughts or to summon up sufficient energy to express them in language.

The patient loses confidence in herself and

will also complain of a lack of decision and will-power. She cannot decide on, nor bring to a satisfactory ending, any desired action, or feels as if she cannot. Even when she has the power to begin to act—for example, reading a book—the effort is soon abandoned, because the same passages are gone over and over again, and before the meaning of a few lines is grasped their connection with the remainder of the passage is forgotten. Often she loses the power of concentrating her attention on anything except her own person.

This enfeeblement of will-power may be shown by an increased general disability. Speaking, writing, walking, eating, answering questions, become increasingly difficult and the patient may become unable to perform the ordinary duties of household life. It is not that these patients are at the moment perverse or wilfully obstinate; rather is it that they cannot will to do these various acts. Sometimes they may tell one that they have really struggled to make up their minds for a particular act but that the effort to overcome the mental hesitation and inertia was futile, and that they could not do it. There is a condition of doubt and an irresolution which is nearly always shown about the simplest details of everyday life. The patient is in constant hesitation from the most trivial motives, with inability to reach any definite result. She worries usually over such trifles as whether she stamped a letter before posting it, whether it was properly addressed, whether she locked a certain door, whether a gas jet is thoroughly turned off, and so on with all the decisions of domestic life.

Some of these patients continually ask questions, especially about their disease. They love to talk of themselves. This is the subject of which they never weary, sometimes the only one on which they can converse. Mental irritability is another common condition. They fret and worry and become ill-tempered and even passionate over mere trifles. If such patients are much to be pitied, those who have the care of them are hardly less so. They require the attention of the entire household, and their shifting moods keep everybody about them in a mingled state of anxious solicitude and resentment.

It often happens that this condition is accompanied by disturbances of the bodily functions, by dyspepsia, palpitations, and insomnia, and consequently some organic disease is feared, when in reality all that is at fault is the nervous functioning.

In extreme cases the patients tire on the slightest effort, and finally they no longer dare walk, either because of the extreme lassitude they feel when erect, or because they suffer from continual giddiness, or because they find the upright position and walking a source of fatigue, uneasiness, and distress. Thenceforward they cease to go out and confine themselves to their room, where they pass the days, seated or more often lying, in complete idleness. In fact all activity is painful to them; they cannot read without becoming tired, nor listen to a conversation of any length; still less can they write, sew, or apply themselves to any other work. They feel vague diffuse pains, the appetite becomes languishing, sometimes the patients grow thin, but often enough they keep up their flesh and have an illusory appearance of comparatively good health.

In some cases there is only a feeling of weight and immobility, but this suffices to make the patient believe that she has lost the use of her limbs. Such loss of power is most common in women who lack those distinct occupations and aims which, in the lives of men, are like the steadying influence of the fly-wheel in an engine. Such patients may remain in bed or on a sofa for months or years, or until some startling incident, or a physician, who understands the nature of the case, restores the powers of motion.

These functional disorders in a minor degree are often found in normal people. We have all experienced these feelings of weakness, but the nervous patient magnifies symptoms and alarms herself. She is sensitive and emotional, and her fatigability is in large part auto-suggested, dependent on a pessimistic state of mind; and that part which is real is aggravated by the emotional fatigue which results from thinking about it. In consequence it will be found that all movements that these patients are told to make seem impossible so long as their attention is fixed on the particular muscles involved in the act, but the movements become easy if the patient's attention is drawn to another muscular group or diverted altogether. This is not the only contradiction. Often we find the same in dyspeptic patients. They may manage a hearty meal one day and the next day they may suffer in spite of the care taken "to eat nothing but light food." Similarly, it is not rare to see headaches disappear by reason of a distraction, or a pleasant visit, even when the patient feared, more than anything else, the fatigue of conversation. On examination we may find many more such contradictions and it is our duty, by an attentive analysis, to separate the kernel of true fatigue from the shell of auto-suggestion.

It is important to make a correct diagnosis: There is the genuine fatigue of nervous exhaustion in women whose health is below par. To this may be added, and frequently exists independently, a memory of fatigability, which has once been experienced, and is evoked more or less continually by auto-suggestion. In the latter case, it is the obsession and not the fatigue which is unhealthy. If one, as a matter of fact, begins any work with a feeling of anxiety or the conviction that it will not go on well, this work will soon become fatiguing, because a mental element has been added to it at the start.

In this form of suggested fatigue, the patient, when she attempts to do anything, usually makes a badly applied effort. For example, walking is a complicated process requiring the adjustment and harmonious working of different groups of muscles, which are in the normal state set in motion by us automatically. Not so in these patients. Their mind is so centred on the setting in motion of cach individual group of tendons and muscles that the movement is retarded, becomes badly adjusted, and causes rapid and severe fatigue. Consequently they collapse readily. Now, let these same patients be influenced by a great emotion, so that their mind is distracted or is centred only in accomplishing the end in view, and they will not only walk but run without the slightest effort or sense of fatigue. I have seen women who complained that walking tired them easily, keep on walking for a considerable length of time without fatigue, while they were talking to someone in whom they were interested or else about their troubles, thus proving that the fatigue experienced is directly proportioned to the degree of consciousness in the effort. The defect in these patients lies in their mentality; they cannot set their muscles in motion with indifference. The very attention which they bring to bear upon the effort that they are making is sufficient to disturb the action which they wish to perform.

In the treatment of such patients we must not confuse the real fatigue, due to loss of nervous energy and which requires physical measures, with the subjective fatigue, for which psychotherapy is the proper remedy. As a rule both forms of fatigue are present, but in a different degree. Real fatigue is greatly exaggerated by the conviction of helplessness and the apprehension concerning all acts which are likely to prove fatiguing; and this conviction and apprehension cause a disharmony of phenomena, that makes the fatigue effective whenever an effort is made.

As regards loss of will-power and mental energy, it is rare among women whose thinking is productive and fertile; but is common among those who let life conquer them, among inactive women of meditative but non-productive brain, and among those who do not work consecutively but in "fits and starts." The one thing that is really trying is the setting in motion. If we do not work regularly, we are constantly obliged to renew the setting in motion, to compel our brain to become attentive, to constrain the intellect to a given task by command, and this even the most gifted find fatiguing.

Loss of memory, indecision, doubts and scruples occur most often in patients who are preoccupied, and who cannot succeed in turning their attention to outside things. Gradually they become convinced of their mental weakness and refuse to make any genuine efforts. This weakness, however, is not due to any lack of psychical efficiency, but is only an indication of the difficulty which a preoccupied patient experiences in fixing the attention on anything but that which is preoccupying her. It is evident that physical measures alone will not cure such patients. What is required is such psychotherapy as will make the preoccupations disappear, when the symptoms which are secondary to them will disappear also. To treat them effectively, we must search for the mental causes in the patient herself and in her environment, and eliminate all sources of worry and emotion, as far as possible. Often a suppressed sorrow or disappointment is the originating cause which has reduced the nervous energy by its constant wear, and the patient will not be well until peace is restored to her mind. Next, calm, judicious reasoning may help; but most important of all is it to draw these patients away from self-contemplation and direct their thoughts into other channels by interesting occupations needing not much exercise.

CHAPTER III

LOSS OF MENTAL CONTROL

MORBID FEARS AND MENTAL DEPRESSION

When nervous debility has persisted for some time, it is not uncommon that there arises a mental symptom which causes the patient considerable distress, namely, either a general feeling of anxiety—a constant but undefined dread of impending danger or misery—or else definite morbid fears. In such a case, the slightest happenings may appear as catastrophes; to any occurrence whatever may be ascribed the least probable and most terrible cause. A woman thus affected will, for example, be overcome by the receipt of a telegram before having learned its contents, or she may read between the lines of a letter most alarming news. She will suffer agonies when her husband is out for a walk or away on a journey, apprehensive that some accident may have befallen him, that he may be ill, or worse still, may have lost his life. If perchance a letter arrives from him later, or he does not return from his walk in time, the agony is still greater and the patient is in absolute despair. Some have the same fear with regard to their son or daughter. Sometimes this dread of accident or disease is so great that abnormal measures of precaution are taken to preserve their safety. Occasionally this fear extends to strangers, so that most ridiculous precautions are taken to protect people who are in no danger whatever.

Morbid fears vary according to the individual. There is no limit to their variety. Not the least trying are those patients who suffer from religious fears, doubts, and scruples. They are generally first seen by their clergymen friends, who, unless they are men of the world, often aggravate the patient's troubles by taking her statements seriously and talking to her freely on religious matters, delighted to have discovered such a devout woman. Fortunately there are many enlightened clergymen to-day who recognise the mental condition of the patient, and, without entering into details with the patient, advise the relatives of her condition and prompt them to consult a physician. Such cases require very careful analysis to discover the primary fear which underlies these religious scruples. Once this primary fear is removed, the patient makes a quick recovery. Such patients are sometimes held to be insane, when actually they are suffering from an obsession due to nervous exhaustion. It often requires expert knowledge to make a diagnosis.

In a large number of cases, certain unreasonable thoughts obtrude themselves and cannot be got rid of by the patient. These so-called OBSESSIONS may consist merely of persistent ideas, harmless in themselves; or they may be emotional in character, when they are very disagreeable and affect the conduct of the person. The latter consist generally of fears, dreads, or aversions, and vary considerably according to the personal experience to which they owe their origin.

One of the commonest fears of this kind is that described as *agoraphobia,* or fear of open places. Such patients dread to cross public squares or wide streets. They dare not leave the house without a companion. Others experience great anxiety when they are compelled to stay in enclosed places, as in rooms with doors and windows closed, so-called *claustrophobia.* If they venture to go to a theatre or concert, or even to a dinner, they must obtain a seat near a door, so that they may leave without a difficulty when the feeling comes over them. Even otherwise strong-minded women can suffer from this complaint. I knew a lady, an expert explorer and mountaineer, free from fear anywhere in the open, not afraid of meeting wild animals, not afraid of disasters on the sea, who could not go to a theatre, her anxiety making her nearly faint.

Some of these sufferers find it intolerable to travel alone in a railway carriage ; others dread to mingle with a crowd. I had a patient who had a great dread of meeting people, at least more than one or two at a time. She could not be induced to go to any public assembly, not even a garden party given by her friends. Yet she was brave under certain circumstances, as she showed one night when there was an alarm of burglars, and she walked out boldly into her garden armed with a gun.

Some patients have an unreasonable fear of fire and must go themselves through the whole house before retiring to bed, visiting every room to ascertain whether all lights and fires are extinguished. This dread is sometimes combined with irresolution and doubt, in which case going through the house once is not sufficient. They begin to doubt whether they have looked properly and go the round several times.

One patient of mine had a dread of burglars. She could not go to sleep without looking under the bed to see whether there was a thief hiding. She took this precaution even when there was not the smallest chance of a stranger entering her premises. The slightest sound during the night was at once interpreted as coming from burglars and caused her to suffer agonies of dread. She hid her valuables in the strangest and most inaccessible places and once forgot where she placed a valuable brooch, of the theft of which she wrongly accused one of her maids. Some months afterwards she discovered it accidentally.

To this category of abnormal fears belongs also the fear which is experienced on ascending a height. Some persons, even at a very slight elevation and when there is no real danger, become giddy and feel as though they will fall, or as though they must throw themselves over.

Similarly, the dread of darkness that so many people have is not cowardice but is due to idiosyncrasy. Much depends on habit in this matter. Most people unaccustomed to sleeping in empty houses experience dreads that come over them when they first try to do it. Every noise is exaggerated in significance; and the creaking of the stairs, and rattling windows and doors, and the wind through the trees, are all made significant of something quite other than what they are.

One of the most curious dreads, very frequently seen and producing more discomfort than could possibly be imagined by anyone who had not seen striking cases of it, is the dread of cats.

A peculiar dread also is that of theft. A lady of my acquaintance confessed to me that she could not enter a shop without having a terror, causing her palpitation and perspiration, that she would be tempted to steal.

These various forms of dread and fear are generally acquisitions caused by some nerve-weakening influence, the absurdity of which is recognised by the victim, but cannot be conquered by her. When the patient has experienced such anxiety on several occasions, then the complaint may become confirmed. She then dreads the anxiety she expects to suffer, and is ill before the actual anxiety does occur; just as people get seasick sometimes before the steamer has begun to move. Hence neither sedatives, tonics, "Weir Mitchell" treatment, nor any other measure will cure a patient who is suffering from morbid fears unless psychotherapy be employed as well, adapted to the individual case.

It is not sufficient, either, for the removal of morbid fears to appeal to the patient's conscious reasoning processes, as the cause of them does not lie there. Most of the fears can be traced to an emotional episode which has been conserved in the unconscious; in a few cases, the original episode has become dissociated. In these states of abnormal fear, when the original experience which caused the fear has become dissociated from consciousness, it is necessary to form a synthesis before a cure can take place. If the dissociated experience is synthetised with consciousness, and thus brought under control and censorship, the attacks may cease.

In other cases, a slow process of re-education of the mental habits and training in mental discipline is required to get rid of these fears and obsessions.

First, we must get rid of the preoccupations of the patient. Then if the phobia refers to something objective, as is the case, for example, with agoraphobia, the patient will be susceptible to re-education. We must reassure her, and show her experimentally that she can master her particular fear by progressively making her accustomed to the various elements of which it is composed. If the phobia depends purely on ideas, as, for instance, the fear of doing harm to self or others, we must explain to the patient the difference between the excess of emotion and the impulse to act; it must be made plain to her that she cannot help feeling apprehension —say—at the sight of knives or an open window for the present, but she need fear no actual harm and will overcome the phobia by practising indifference as to the consequences. The sight of the knives will then still bring up in the memory associated ideas for some time; but gradually they will lose their emotional significance, and in a short time she will be able to handle these instruments without any apprehension.

It is important to proceed cautiously, more by making the patient forget her fears than by arousing a mental struggle. If the patient can be made to learn to view with indifference the possibility of an accident, she will recover very quickly. The soldier in battle does not think of the injuries he is likely to receive; his mind is entirely centred on the destruction of the enemy. He would be useless as a fighting machine if he were preoccupied with his own person. Similarly, the patients in question must learn to manifest their will-power without the retarding influence of anxious emotions. The woman suffering from agoraphobia must be made to walk first only a few steps, and gradually longer distances to the shops or houses she intends to visit, centring her mind on the execution of the act or diverting her attention altogether. The first success will reassure her. I further impress upon the patient the fact that if she will observe closely all the objects she sees on her walk, if she will, so to say, "throw out" her mind, she will prevent introspection and preoccupation and forget her fear. We must also create new ideas for the patient and new associations of ideas, to overlay and blot out the old phobic ideas. Needless to say, that not only each variety of fear, but each case requires individual treatment; and all we can do here is merely to indicate the general lines on which it should be conducted.

The limited self-control of these patients often leads to IMPULSIVE ACTIONS, which may be merely useless or absurd acts, or more or less dangerous ones leading to injury or theft. When the act is completed the patient experiences a peculiar satisfaction and later a feeling of remorse followed by anxiety lest the act be repeated. In such a case of *kleptomania*, as distinguished from thieving, the articles taken are usually not made use of or replaced unawares. It is the shame of beïng regarded as a thief that prevents a frank confession. Often, as already mentioned, there is only a *fear* of stealing.

HYPOCHONDRIASIS. We all of us get tired; the human mechanism is so complicated that hardly a day goes by without our noticing some creaking in the works; sometimes it is gastric trouble, or a slight pain or palpitation of the heart, or a transient neuralgia. We know what it is and as a rule are not upset about it. The nervous person, however, is easily frightened; she regards her weariness and discomforts with great concern, and makes them last longer by the attention she pays to herself.

In some women there is such a morbid anxiety as to health and such exaggerated, if not illusory, ideas as to the existence of certain bodily diseases, that attention becomes concentrated upon it and physical sensibility exalted; with the result that passing physical sensations or slight ailments eventually assume to the deluded imagination a grave and ominous character. There is an apprehension or fear of disease, not a genuine conviction, hence the patient talks to everyone she meets about her ailments to get some further clues in regard to their realities. At first she will be amenable to reason; but if not dealt with firmly, and if the nervous exhaustion which lies at the root of her trouble is not properly treated, her fear may give way to a fixed idea. Still there is no real physical disease; the ailment is in reality a spiritual infirmity. Such subjects generally lead sedentary and solitary lives, and their morbidity is often intensified by reading quack literature. In most of them, there has been an unhealthy mental attitude or want of object in life that has made them preoccupied with self, their own comforts and discomforts, sensations and feelings.

There is often a state of MENTAL GLOOM and DEPRESSION, but, unlike the melancholic woman, the patient does not brood unoccupied and alone over her miseries, but is constantly willing and even eager to pour out her miseries to those about her. It is certainly true that to tell one's troubles is often a help and relief; but frequently the husband or friends of the patient are too loving and indulgent and allow the patient to talk too much of her mental and bodily ills. Such repetition helps to fix them in her mind, to intensify them, often really makes them worse; and even when it does not do this, it is very likely to suggest an unconscious exaggeration to make a good round tale, and from this to imagining symptoms is a short and sadly easy step. Moreover, this talking creates a desire for more sympathy; the invalid wants more and more of it, and if the real ailments do not furnish ground for complaint, they may readily be magnified. There are patients who literally "take it out" of everyone near, to the latter's detriment yet not to their own gain. An ordinary quarter of an hour's visit to such patients leaves one exhausted, squeezed dry. They use up nurses like a machine grinding material. I have seen charming people of this sort, intellectual, cultivated, with lively sympathies of their own, who are quite unable to appreciate their peculiar influence upon others; and cannot understand why no companion or nurse will stay longer than she can help.

Not for a moment should this be taken as meaning that loving service and earnest affection are not valuable and helpful to these patients—but they must be mingled with intelligence, with real comprehension, and there must be a certain detached and critical position maintained in order to keep the judgment unimpaired. True sympathy keeps its ability to hold the balance between over-indulgence of whims, permitting the growth of fanciful troubles, encouraging complaints, on the one side, and neglect or want of recognition of the actual state of the patient on the other. It must be remembered that the sufferings of the hypochondriacal woman are legitimate sufferings, quite as legitimate as if they were due to some affected organ. She may exaggerate her sufferings, but this is sometimes true even for patients who are organically afflicted; for the pain, which is a purely subjective phenomenon, is felt in proportion to the attention that is brought to bear upon it.

Distraction, getting the mind away from the trouble, the simple therapeutic action of explanation and reassurance, and re-education without making the patient aware of it, are the methods of treatment that should be employed.

MELANCHOLIA. Sometimes people suffer not from definite fears, but from indefinite fears of impending evil; a fear of something, they do not know what. This morbid anxiety and groundless apprehension occurs most often in women descended from a neuropathic stock; and the exciting cause is frequently exhaustion, particularly after childbirth, or produced in a delicate woman by prolonged suckling, or at the "change of life." It occurs equally often in spinsters; indeed, it can occur in any woman of a nervous, hypersensitive temperament. Women of this temperament feel pleasure more keenly, but they also tend to feel pain intensely, whether it be of physical or mental origin, when depressing events occur.

A healthy woman may, indeed, experience sudden shocks, griefs, fears, and apprehensions; but she reasons with them until her misery becomes abated, the pangs of grief are mitigated, consolation is felt, and new interests and aspirations are awakened. Such depression is of short duration, does not impair the reasoning power, does not greatly interfere with self-control, or with the general nutrition of the body. In some women—those of a neuropathic stock—this is not so. The patient feels sad, out of spirits, cannot explain the reason for her depression or divest herself of it. Her grief becomes protracted and deepened, and she will not be comforted. A state of unyielding moody misery becomes habitual; the patient complains of insomnia, or that the sleep is broken by unpleasant dreams, and is unrefreshing. The subject is often acutely conscientious, and distresses herself needlessly about family matters. She may appreciate the unreasonableness of her depression, but she cannot rid herself of it. Her attention is riveted to painful impressions and cannot be attracted by outward allurements. Moreover, the voluntary power is impaired so that the patient is deprived of resolution and the power of decision. Her will is paralysed, and she may be so inactive that she will not move unless obliged to do so. There is a disinclination for work, an indifference to the ordinary interests of life, and a desire for seclusion. Amusements are a nuisance to her. She finds even letter-writing a bore, and is often irritable to those about her in a way she never was previously. This retardation applies to all actions; she moves slowly, hesitates over everything, and appears to think slowly. She can find no pleasure in anything, everything has become irksome; nor can she be touched by the misfortune of others, her own distress absorbing her whole attention.

Her intellect is intact, but the ideas seem unable to flow. She is incapable of long-sustained mental effort. Former pursuits and studies become distasteful or are altogether abandoned. She is desperately unhappy. She may weep and sob a great deal and wish she were dead.

It is very important to distinguish organic depression—melancholia—from purely functional depression. Mistakes are frequently made.

Whenever such undue depression occurs, the friends of the patient should be on their guard and take early steps to consult their family physician. Taken in time, a speedy recovery is almost certain; if neglected, the depression may become chronic and the prospects of a cure become more and more remote. Some of these patients develop true delusions, as, for instance, the conviction that they have cancer of the stomach, or the conviction of having a serpent in the intestines. They are not simply apprehensive or doubtful, they are convinced.

CHAPTER IV

HEADACHE, NEURALGIA, AND OTHER PAINS

IN some patients it is not so much lassitude and fatigue that they suffer from than a general HYPERSENSITIVENESS, which is still more annoying. The ordinary impressions made during everyday life upon the senses, which to the healthy individual are pleasant or indifferent, or at any rate easily tolerable, become obtrusive evils, while the well-meant efforts of friends, often in the direction of social entertainment and amusement, are so many sources of irritation. Uncomfortable sensations, discomforts, sense of unequal pressure or of constriction may occur in every part of the body. When the special senses are involved, the eye is extremely sensitive to light, and hearing is markedly exaggerated, so that the slightest sound, such as the rustling of a newspaper, is annoying, and the ticking of a watch, not to say of a clock, may be extremely distressing.

If such patients are asked whether they are nervous, they are often indignant at the question; though they readily own that they cannot bear the slightest noise or a domestic upset, and that they are over-sensitive to emotional stimuli. Temper may not be easily ruffled; but they are ready to jump "out of their skin" at the jarring of a door, and are in agony at hearing the sound of footsteps overhead. It is torture to some to hear others converse; others say that on the most trivial occurrence they "feel all of a tremble, all of a shake."

The state of mind such patients get into is well illustrated by the following case of a lady who, consequent on some family trouble, had a nervous breakdown, showing itself chiefly by hypersensibility. The closing of doors in her house, the twittering of birds in her garden, the ringing of glasses carried on a tray, the dropping of even a light article, creaking boots, etc., all noises, however slight, whether real or anticipated, caused her intense agony and irritability. She took rooms in a quiet house and on enquiry on the next morning how she had slept she replied: "Not at all; I heard a door bang just before retiring to bed, and I could not go to sleep for fear a door might bang again."

From hypersensitiveness it is a short step to actual PAIN, especially in people who lack definite occupation and a serious purpose in life and are given to habits of introspection. By concentration of mind on a particular portion of the body the ordinary functions of that part, usually accomplished quite unconsciously, become first a source of uneasy discomfort and then an ache or pain. There are many nervous people whose susceptibility to pain has been so much increased by their lack of self-control, and their tendency to react easily to pain, that even slight pain has become a torment. In most cases nothing is found locally, or at most there is some functional disturbance so slight that, though it may be felt by a great many people, others do not complain of it at all. It seems evident, therefore, that the discomfort must result from the sensitiveness of the individual emphasising the significance of some slight disturbance. While such pain is often spoken of as imaginary, it must be remembered that this does not mean that it is non-existent. On the contrary, it may be much more real to the patient than physical ailment.

HEADACHE is unquestionably one of the most common of all common ailments. It exists among all classes of society. It occurs much more frequently in women than in men. It is complained of particularly by those who have little regular occupation and no serious absorbing interest in life. There are many women of leisure who have regular headaches for which they must have some remedy at hand or the pain becomes intolerable; but there are few women strenuously occupied with business affairs or with interests in which their attention is absorbed who find themselves under any such necessity. Of many women one might say: once a headache, always a headache. They do not take the trouble to consult a physician to ascertain and remove the cause, but fly to any quack remedy which gives them temporary relief. Any number of headache cures are advertised in the daily papers, in the street cars, on the signboards, even in medical journals; and besides these nearly every druggist has his own special preparation for headache, so it would seem as though literally many millions of doses of these headache cures must be taken every week.

It is rare that the cause of the headache is mental overwork; usually it is the worry and anxiety and dread over the work that is being done that is the source. There are of course organic headaches due to definite pathological conditions; but the great majority of headaches complained of are the result of anxiety and worry concerning money affairs, conduct of children, love affairs, and other emotional factors, together with over-attention to certain sensations and queer feelings about the head, some of them normal, some of them only slightly abnormal, which are annoyances rather than pain, but which emphasised by concentration of attention on them become a torment. The pain varies in intensity, from the slight, which merely inconveniences, to the agonising pain sufficient to prostrate the patient, and make her lie by for some days.

The symptoms vary somewhat when it is purely a *nervous headache* and when a nervous headache is associated with an anæmic, hyperæmic, or toxic condition of the blood. It is common for nervous patients to suffer from various more or less distressing sensations in the head, which have not the character of actual pain. The sensations vary in different cases; but by far the most frequent is a sense of pressure, sometimes trifling, sometimes as if a heavy weight were on the head. Its common seat is at the top of the head, but it is sometimes felt in other situations. A sensation of heat or burning is sometimes described. A vague sense of fulness is not uncommon, and it is at times accompanied by a sense of throbbing. Many other annoying sensations in this region are also complained of, notably a feeling as if the scalp were drawn tightly over the skull or as if it were encompassed by a constricting band. Sometimes patients speak of a feeling of weight in the head or that the brain feels dead; they say that they cannot think and are in agony for fear of losing their reason. Others state that they felt something give way in their brain, that something "snapped," and they have never been the same since. It is important to note that practically all these feelings, whether they appear to emanate from the scalp or from within the skull, are increased by mental application.

In *anæmic* women, headache arises from a deficiency of blood within the cranial cavity. Sometimes those affected by this variety of headache complain of a sensation of tightness about the forehead; sometimes again the pain is more restricted in character and manifests itself in clawing sensations, which are particularly well marked at the vertex. Whatever the location of the pain may be, it is almost invariably less pronounced when the subject is in the recumbent position than when the body is maintained in an erect attitude. Less pain is therefore felt during the latter part of the night and early morning than during the day. In the more extreme cases the simple act of rising is sufficient to cause giddiness and fainting.

In *full-blooded* women the headache is due to congestion giving a sensation of fulness, as though the cranium were too small for its contents. As a rule the painful sensations are not circumscribed in character, but are distributed throughout the entire extent of the cranium. The pain is constant, and is augmented by assuming the recumbent posture; consequently sleep is more or less profoundly affected. All forms of mental or physical exertion are followed by exacerbation of pain accompanied by more or less giddiness. The subject is extremely irritable and aroused to inordinate passion by the most trivial circumstance, is pessimistic, depressed, and lachrymose, and inclined to find fault with all about her.

Migraine, sick, or bilious headache comes on in paroxysms. The pain is seldom absent and may exist alone, but it is commonly accompanied by nausea and vomiting, and it is often preceded by some disorder of the sense of sight. The symptoms are frequently one-sided. Women suffer from migraine more frequently than men. Its occurrence is generally related to influences that depress and weaken the nervous system, either directly or through the general health. Fatigue and excitement are the most common. Digestive disturbance is sometimes mentioned as a cause, and in some cases a particular article of diet will always induce an attack. Over-stimulation of the eyes may also bring on an attack, as after visiting a cinematograph show or a tour round a picture gallery. When the attacks consist of simple headache the patient often wakes up with it. The face gets pale and "pinched."

Toxic headache is a form of headache caused by some chemical change in the constitution of the blood. The nature of the pains arising from toxic causes is variable in character. Sometimes the subject complains of a heavy, dull sensation in the head, which may or may not be accompanied by giddiness; or the pain is sharp and is described as splitting or boring. According to the extent of the intoxication, the faculties of the mind are more or less affected. There may be actual delirium, as in violent febrile disturbances, or the only symptoms noticed are heaviness and slight mental confusion.

In headache, as in other ailments, the first duty is to ascertain the cause. Many headaches have a definite exciting cause, which can be removed, with the result that the patient is permanently cured. A thorough examination of the various systems of the body and the special senses will be necessary. As already pointed out, however, few headaches are really so severe as described by the patients. What has happened is that a simple pathological condition has been exaggerated by over-attention, and the symptoms may persist even when the physical cause is no longer operative. Besides providing for distraction of mind, and teaching mental discipline, we may have to change the habits of the patient. Some women are so disorderly in their personal arrangements, and in all that pertains to their business or household, that all work requires an extraordinary effort and their worries are increased tenfold. No wonder that they are constantly subject to mental strain and suffer as a consequence from headache. Others are irregular in their meals, often take insufficient food or go without for a considerable time, or live almost entirely on tea and coffee, with the result that their head feels uncomfortable. A little more regularity and orderliness would prevent these attacks.

In certain cases, particularly in purely nervous headache, the application of a weak galvanic current to the affected regions of the head removes the pain, in many instances almost instantaneously. The patients declare that the head feels lighter, the ideas are clearer, there is greater power of attention; it is as if a weight had been removed from the brain. This improvement is more marked after each application, until cure is complete. Of course, this success may be due as much to suggestion as to the power of the electricity; but, after careful observation, I feel convinced that electricity has undoubtedly a beneficial effect, owing to its influence on the circulation and on the brain itself.

NOISES IN THE HEAD are often complained of by nervous patients. In many cases these are due to variations in the quantity, quality, and pressure of the blood, either in the ear itself or in the brain, such as are induced in adults by worry, excitement, fatigue, debility, or indigestion. These noises are either ringing, whistling, hissing, cracking, pulsating, blowing, continuous or intermittent. All these sounds may be absent, and yet the subject may still be greatly annoyed by hearing the beat of the pulse in her ear when the head is on the pillow. Of course, noises in the head are frequently associated with some disease in the ear, but with noises arising from this cause we are not here concerned.

Nothing more painful or harder to bear can be imagined than continual noises in the head. They are apt to depress the tone of the mind and of the whole nervous system of the unfortunate sufferer. The enjoyment of life is destroyed, the temper soured, and the power of work greatly reduced. It is seldom that patients get accustomed to the noise in their ears, and are able to follow the advice so freely tendered to them by their friends, that they should forget all about it and think of something else; on the contrary, in the large majority of cases no amusement or change of occupation and scene has the slightest influence upon it, and the trouble is felt as keenly after it has lasted for years as it was when it first began.

There is perhaps no other complaint so distressing and at the same time so difficult to treat. The method that I have found the most successful is that of "suggestion." By suggestion treatment, we get the patient to focus her thoughts so well on whatever she has in hand that she ceases to dread the noises, and gradually learns to disregard them. The noises then frequently disappear; but if they do still persist they are no longer exaggerated, and it is then easier to discover their true cause and to attend to them by the proper physical measures.

Backache is another source of great distress and suffering to women. The spine is tender to pressure, and in severe cases this tenderness may extend over its entire length. It may be so acute that even the weight of the clothing is unbearable, and the sufferer cannot sit down without an air cushion under her. In cases of lesser severity, the upper and lower extremities of the spine may alone be sensitive, and from the latter situation the sensitiveness may extend into the hips. There may be disinclination to move or twist the body, but not so marked as in lumbago, sprain, or more serious and deeper troubles. It is very important that an accurate diagnosis should be made. The intensity of the pain varies from a very slight one, which does not prevent moving about, to one which, for a time, usurps the place of all other sensations, confining women to their bed for a few days. The pain is usually provoked by slight fatigue. The patients tire very readily; after slight physical exertion, a short walk, ascending a single flight of stairs, standing for a short length of time, they are compelled to retire to bed. The pain is almost always fugitive in the upper portions of the spine, and principally settles in its lower extremity, radiating to the small of the back, the loins, thighs, and legs. The pain is generally described as an aching or numbing pain, a gnawing, dragging, burning, or grinding pain; a sensation as if the back were broken, or as if it were opening and shutting. There is usually a high degree of mental irritability. Local treatment, gentle, simple, yet directed with the proper therapeutic purpose so as to create a favourable expectancy in the patient's mind, will do much for this condition.

NEURALGIA is an affection of the nerves, the chief characteristic of which is severe and sudden pain occurring in one or more nerve trunks and radiating towards the periphery. In many patients the neuralgic tendency is deeply rooted; they suffer from neuralgia first in one situation and then in another during the course of years. The first attack is always preceded by a condition of debility, an impairment of the general health, resulting from general or special causes: overwork of mind or body, prolonged fatigue, anæmia of every degree and causation, and especially exposure to cold. The disease is liable to occur in persons of a nervous temperament, persons easily excitable, irritable, or anxious and worrying over the trifling ills of life. Patients suffering from rheumatism and gout are predisposed to it. Neuralgic pains are also common in hysteria.

The onset of the disease is usually heralded by vague muscular twitchings or sensations of pricking, quickly succeeded by evanescent darting pains. The pains are recurrent in character, and succeed each other with ever increasing frequency and intensity until, in the more severe attacks, the patient suffers the most excruciating agony. Sometimes the pains are described as resembling the sensations produced by the prick of red-hot needles; other subjects complain that they feel as though they were being lacerated with a saw, or as if electric sparks were projected along the course of their nerves. These pains are sometimes stationary, and are ascribed by the subject to particular districts, which are found to correspond to the course of a nerve trunk. At other times they are ambulatory and dart from place to place. The most common forms of neuralgia are *facial neuralgia* and *sciatica.*

Neuralgia, of whatever variety, requires constitutional as well as local remedies, according to the cause which originated it. As regards local applications, neuralgia is even more readily influenced than headache by the application of galvanism to the affected nerve. Such, at all events, is my personal experience. Of late, since the introduction of radium, radium-ionisation has given splendid results even in chronic cases, where the pain could previously be mitigated only by opium or morphia. I have known the pain to disappear at the first application in idiopathic neuralgia without the assistance of drugs, administered either by mouth or locally. When this is not the case we may be sure that the fault lies largely, if not entirely, in the mental condition of the patient.

Of all the misfortunes which a human being may suffer, the most striking and the most obtrusive is certainly pain. Loss of wealth may be forgotten, loss of strength may matter but little, but pain cannot be put aside. It cannot be forgotten and it becomes an obsession, for it denies the claim of the mind to consider aught else. Pain may be created by the concentration of the mind on a particular part of the body, rendering that part hypersensitive. For example, if we try and think of the big toe for some length of time, we shall experience queer feelings in it. But besides originating pain, the mind is still more powerful in increasing pain that exists from one cause or another, so that slight discomforts may be made insupportable. Individuals differ very much as regards the tolerance of pain. What seems unendurable to many may be little more than passing annoyance to others.

Over-sensitive patients must be trained to bear discomfort for a while until their mind is diverted to other things from the concentration of attention on those functions which is causing their disturbance. Pain differs also according to circumstances. What would be under ordinary circumstances intolerable torture, especially to sensitive people, may, because of intense preoccupation of mind, remain absolutely unnoticed. For instance, in the excitement of a panic people may suffer what would, under other conditions, be excruciating agony, and yet not know they are hurt. To a woman without serious interests even slight pain, if continuous, may be unbearable, and is often made worse by complaining about it and resisting it. Were she calmly to accept the pain as a matter of fact, it would be immediately robbed of one-half its torture. Pain has always been dreaded, but it seems as if with the increase of comfort its terrors have increased. Many pains could be easily borne were it not for the worry and dread that accompany them. What these patients need is occupation that really catches their interest and takes attention from themselves, and they require training in self-control. It is the dread of pain which tempts so many patients to the use of drugs, which do serious harm, and for which a habit is easily acquired. The removal of the cause is the only true method of the removal of pain. To drown a pain by drugs, to obtund the parts so that no pain is felt, is to throw away the warning which the pain has given. Only when the removal of the cause is beyond human skill may we content ourselves with mere relief of pain.

CHAPTER V

INSOMNIA

Among the symptoms of nervous disorder, there is one of great importance by reason of its frequency and the aggravation of the patient's condition that it causes. This is insomnia. On the whole, women suffer less frequently from sleeplessness, and can bear the loss of sleep better than men. The length of time they can devote themselves to night-nursing in response to the calls of affection or duty has scarcely any limit. On the other hand, many women's work is rather monotonous; they are seldom in the open air and take little exercise, which causes combined are not conducive to good sleep.

Sleep varies in degree and kind from the slight to the profound. It may be tranquil; it may be disturbed; it may be short or it may be prolonged. Sleep is as necessary to the human economy as air is to respiration and vitality. It is as natural for us to sleep every twenty-four hours, as it is for the earth to turn upon its axis. Sleep favours nutrition, and nutrition is essential to sleep. Sleep equalises the balance of power between the automatic and the volitional. This balance of power is essential to sleep. Want of sleep will in time wear out the finest and strongest brain. All sorts of nervous disorders result from want of sleep. Of course, as in everything else, the widest differences may be observed between one person and another in regard to the amount of sleep required. There are adults who do not require more than five and a half to seven hours, and there are others who take nine hours and over. No general rule can be laid down to cover all cases. Much depends on the nature of occupation and on habit. The habit of sleeping too little is less frequent among women than that of sleeping too much. Many women allow themselves an altogether unnecessary quantity of sleep, and are dissatisfied unless they secure a really abnormal allowance. On the other hand, there are some women with very active brains who sleep very little, and enjoy good health up to old age, if they live otherwise correctly. As a rule, anæmic and nervous women recuperate with extreme slowness and require ten hours or more of sleep properly to redress the balance. As a rough working average, it may be stated that the majority of healthy women require about eight hours of sleep. As a rule, it is not the length of sleep, but the quality, which is at fault.

Many nervous people sleep well, just as some eat well; it is probable that the ability to do either or both of these acts saves them from worse nervousness at least. Many people get more sleep than they are willing to admit. Thus the hypochondriacal woman whose fancy runs this way will woefully assert that she only gets four or five hours' sleep. It is sometimes necessary to prove conclusively to a patient that more sleep is secured than she supposes. One good plan is to suggest to the patient, who says she "never closed an eye all night," to sit up all night. She will find she cannot do it, and will then generally admit that she must after all have slept a good deal.

Patients sometimes describe their sleep at night as abnormally profound; but complain that they are so little refreshed by it that they remain drowsy and lethargic during the day, unable to attend to business, and fall asleep after making the slightest effort. Sustained attention becomes impossible, even if the drowsiness is not succeeded by real sleep. *Drowsiness* is the opposite condition to insomnia and sleeplessness, and is equally a sign of nervous exhaustion. Such patients, when asked if they sleep, will sometimes answer, " Yes, I can sleep night and day."

The majority of patients suffering from nervousness, sleep badly, but their insomnia appears under very different forms. There are patients who get to sleep with difficulty. They go to bed tired, but when they are in bed sleep does not come. Some recognise the fact that they are kept awake by obsessions which they try in vain to get rid of. Others state that their thoughts are not fixed on any disturbing subject, but that they cannot fall asleep. Certain patients fall asleep easily, but they wake up at the end of a few hours and cannot get to sleep again ; many fall asleep toward morning at the hour when they ought to get up.

In those waking periods noises, habitually disregarded by the healthy, obtrude themselves upon the notice of the patient. The sounds of passing vehicles, the striking of clocks, the barking of dogs, all accentuated by the prevailing silence, keep the patient in a condition of annoyed expectancy. Pillows and mattresses are found to be too hard or not hard enough. Each position reveals a sensitive area, and every change of position yet another. The brain is in a whirl, and the thoughts dwell chiefly on the anxieties and disagreeable aspects of life.

Insomnia is frequently associated with morbid fears, and is sometimes their direct consequence. The feeling of alarm keeps the patient awake, or so blends with her dreams that sleep is taken only in brief snatches. Dyspeptic troubles, palpitation of the heart, sensations of flushing, and cutaneous irritations, a feeling which can only be described as one of fidgetiness, or inability to keep still, are often superadded to the morbid dread, and tend to make sleep impossible. Such patients are kept awake by the discomforts or pains they suffer; when relieved of them, they are able to sleep.

Sleep is often prevented by depressing emotions, anxiety, or excitement. At the present day, when so many people, either from choice or necessity, spend their time in passing from one form of excitement to another, when such an enormous amount of work or play has to be got through in a limited number of hours, it is not to be wondered at that sleeplessness is so common a trouble, or that specifics for its relief should be so eagerly sought after and so recklessly employed. In some cases, comparatively slight causes are sufficient to render the individual sleepless, especially if they operate late in the day.

Others sleep, but with agitated sleep, disturbed by dreams and nightmares. Sometimes they preserve no memory of the dream, but are conscious of having had an interrupted and disturbed sleep, and they state in the morning that they have not rested well. All we can say of dreams is that, when not arising from external stimulation, such as uncovering of the bedclothes, or internal organic sensations, such as discomfort or pain, they are due, to put it crudely, to different areas of the brain or tissues and parts of the body varying in the degree of their fatigue, and consequently in the soundness of their sleep. The dream may consist of distorted waking experiences, and is frequently the subconscious expression of ardent desires or antecedent doubts, scruples and anxieties. In sleep, the censorship of the normal waking consciousness is removed, the suppressed or dissociated experiences gain the upper hand and, coloured by the imagination, they form new combinations resulting in a weird phantasmagoria. The troubled or horrid dreams which occur during sickness are probably due to the toxins with which the blood is loaded, torturing the brain areas, in which the images conjured up are stored. Similarly, the gruesome visions and nightmares which embitter the slumbers of those under the stress of violent emotions and mental suffering are due to similar action of the fatigue-poisons produced by these states. While perfectly normal sleep is dreamless, yet a moderate amount of dreaming, especially if the images evoked are of a pleasing or indifferent character, is quite compatible with good and refreshing slumber. Persistent or frequent bad dreams are, like insomnia, a sign of ill-health, and should be regarded and treated as such.

A highly annoying incident in connection with sleep among nervous patients is "starting" in sleep. It occasionally happens that just when a patient is dozing off, she suddenly starts and, almost before she realises it, she is fully awake, her heart beating emphatically and there may even be a little feeling of oppression on the chest. The thought that this forcible beat of the heart must mean some serious pathological condition will obtrude itself on many people, and if it does, sleep is sure to be disturbed. At times this starting from sleep seems due to some unusual noise. In certain nervous states, even slight noises produce an exaggerated reaction. Any of the small noises that sound so loud in the stillness of the night may serve to wake the patient so thoroughly after a preliminary doze that sleep is disturbed for some time. As a rule, however, such noises would not disturb people if they were in normal healthy condition, or at least the disturbance would be only momentary. It is much more a question of personal sensitiveness and anxious expectancy and over-irritability than anything else.

The first duty of the physician is to remove the cause of sleeplessness. Supposing he fails in this, either because he cannot ascertain it or because on account of circumstances the cause is not removable, then he must choose such agencies as will combat the difficulty. In any case, the physician should first insist on a few simple rules, which every woman suffering from insomnia can carry out for herself.

The one procedure which most universally disposes to sound sleep is one which is within the reach of all, and that is getting well tired.

Another rule is to practise going to bed at a definite hour every night and getting up at a definite time every morning; moreover, to get up immediately on waking. It is well known that the functions of the body are performed rhythmically, and by training ourselves to definite time for sleeping, and avoiding all exciting causes prior to going to bed, sleep is almost sure to come. All our functions are regulated by habit. We often have an appetite at the hour for dinner, even when we have not spent our strength or exhausted our capital, and even when we have taken food a few hours before. Our eyelids grow heavy at the time when we habitually go to bed, even though we have displayed no particular activity during the daytime; and when we are accustomed to going to bed late, we cannot go to sleep, although by reason of hard, physical, or mental work we may be so tired that we are ready to say: "I can do no more."

Another essential to procure refreshing sleep is to undress the body and undress the mind, to remove the traces of the day's toil from the face and hands, at least, and the traces of the day's cares from the soul; to brush the hair and arrange it in such a way that it will not interfere with an easy position of the head, and to brush from one's thoughts the things that annoy, by refusing to let them occupy the centre of consciousness. When I speak of undressing the mind, I mean, therefore, to lay aside cares, to withdraw interest from the external world, and so allow the higher brain centres to become inactive. To this end, it is not well to prolong one's work and cares up to the hour of retiring. Hard work fatigues us, but it does not make us sleepy. The questions that have absorbed us during the day have a vicious way of cropping up in our minds at night, do what we will to drive them out. We are fatigued through and through, but we are painfully wide awake. I therefore impress upon my patients to have done with all serious thoughts before entering their bedroom. None but cheering and soothing reflections, if any, should take place prior to going to bed. Any topic which stimulates the brain to great activity, whether intellectually or emotionally, must be carefully excluded. There should be a period of absolute quiet before retiring to bed.

There is one preoccupation which is especially dangerous; it is that of sleep itself. A great deal of the insomnia of nervous patients originates in, and is fostered by, an obstinate and continued belief that sleep is impossible. When one does not sleep and is impatient because one does not sleep, and keeps turning over and over, and growing more and more vexed, one creates a state of agitation which hinders sleep. Many patients approach the night with a fixed idea that they will not sleep, and spend their time reckoning the unhappy consequences which this night of insomnia will have for their well-being on the morrow. They count the bad nights which they have already had, persuaded that this one will follow in line and resemble the others.

To dissipate these phobias which prevent the mind from attaining its necessary calm, I have been accustomed to tell my patients: "Sleep is like a pigeon. It comes to you if you have the appearance of not looking for it; it flies away if you try to catch it." The patient must lose all fear of insomnia. For this purpose, she should approach the question of sleep with a perfect indifference which may be summed up in this idea: "If I sleep, so much the better; if I do not sleep, it does not matter either!" It is only when the mental vibration ceases that sleep comes by itself.

Except invalids, no person should lie in bed during the morning hours when not asleep. Even when awake in the middle of the night and unable to sleep, I have advised getting up and doing some simple non-exciting mechanical work for half an hour or so rather than remaining fidgety in bed. Getting up under these circumstances soon produces a tired feeling, and the body being cooled a little, the warmth of the bed is again appreciated, and sleep is more likely to follow.

Many people can read themselves to sleep with some light novel or magazine. Others, particularly those who suffer from eye-strain, find themselves wider awake the more they read, even though the reading is of the lightest character.

In order to sleep well, patients must be thoroughly comfortable in bed. Most people find they sleep easiest with a reasonably firm pillow, not too low, so that the head is a little higher than the body; others raise the head of the bed, so that there is a gentle slope. The lateral position is to be preferred to lying on the back. Sensitive persons sometimes obtain sleep by changing their position in bed, or, better still, the position of the bed. It is held by some to be of great importance whether the bed faces North, South, East, or West. Others sleep when they have a change of room, and others when they have a change of air.

In patients who suffer from agitated nerves or mental excitement, sleep is sometimes secured by taking a bath before going to bed at a temperature of 99 or 100 degrees Fahrenheit, that is to say, a little above the temperature of the body, and staying in it for fifteen or twenty minutes. This procedure has the effect of allaying tho nervous irritability.

Diet has little influence on sleep; except in so far as food, unsuitable in kind or the time when it is taken, may produce disturbances of digestion and through these of the general balance of health. It is difficult to get sleep on "an empty stomach," or, at least, when the stomach has been empty so long that gnawing and hunger are felt. The processes of digestion probably go on more slowly during sleep, but they are perfectly carried out, as is illustrated by the almost invariable habit among animals of going to sleep directly after a meal. Indeed, a moderate amount of food in the stomach or intestines seems to promote slumber. Many night-workers, for instance, sleep much better for taking a light supper or a glass of hot milk with a biscuit just before retiring. At the same time, an overloaded stomach is not conducive to refreshing sleep, although that condition makes one drowsy.

What most people forget is that there must be a cause for their sleeplessness. There is no such thing as uncaused sleeplessness any more than there is uncaused loss of appetite, of strength, or weight. All of them are signals of trouble and should be promptly regarded and investigated as such. We may have to remedy digestive derangements to relieve local irritations, to correct disturbances of circulation, to relieve anæmia and debilitated conditions, and to secure due regard to sanitary requirements.

Many a woman who works all day in an ill-ventilated room and takes little or no exercise, or who slaves over her housework or her needlework or embroidery and almost forgets that there is such a thing as open air, many a woman who is in the early stage of some disease, when she finds that she cannot sleep, instead of regarding it as nature's danger signal, demanding investigation and change of habits, swallows some sleeping draught and persists in her suicidal course until a breakdown results, that she can no longer shut her eyes to. Drugs for the sake of sleep should never be taken except upon the advice and with the knowledge of a physician who is acquainted with the general conditions under which the person is living. Self-administered drugs are especially dangerous to the nervous person whose moral courage and self-control are at fault; they easily fall victims to the drug habit. A great many people do not take the trouble to think into the matter as far as that. All they want is to get the immediate result; and if this can be done through a drug, they make the venture.

The sleeplessness, which is so distressing and exhausting, is often only an expression of the nervous irritability and obsessions of the sufferer. To temporarily drown one's sensibilities with narcotics is a sure way of intensifying the condition which it should be our endeavour to remedy in some more rational manner. Narcotics have their place in medicine like other poisonous drugs, but that place is becoming steadily smaller as cases are more painstakingly and intelligently studied. There are many which produce a state of unconsciousness resembling sleep, and some of these are unfortunately much resorted to for this purpose. Though permissible in skilled hands, their habitual use is dangerous, both because they are all poisons—weak ones, it is true, but true poisons, and because they smother the symptom without doing anything to relieve the diseased condition which caused it.

I have never experienced any difficulty in inducing sleep without the aid of drugs, even in patients who suffered from acute pains due to organic disease. The probability is that, whatever the circumstance, there is something mentally in the patient's subconscious sphere which keeps her awake; and therefore it is by mental influence that we must overcome the insomnia. I cannot explain otherwise the wonderful and immediate results achieved by psychotherapy, considering too, that the psychotherapist's services are rarely called for until all other remedies have failed. In what this psychic power consists, it is difficult to say, nor is there any one method. I can only say that probably success depends a great deal on the personality of the physician, on his knowledge of mind and character, his sympathy for human talents, virtues, and failings, and his ability to establish instantaneously and intuitively a bond between himself and the patient.

Obstinate cases often do well by the application of mild galvanic currents. I have found the effects to be not only temporary, but permanent. The immediate relief is decidedly great, the permanent improvement is developed gradually and slowly, and results from the general influence of the electricity upon the nervous system.

CHAPTER VI

NERVOUS DYSPEPSIA

It is no exaggeration to say that there is hardly one person suffering from nervous disorder whose digestion does not become affected sooner or later. Indigestion is a common complaint amongst nervous women. Most of them err on the side of eating too little than eating too much, and the little food they take is often not nourishing. Very few women take an intelligent interest in what they eat. Anything will do, they say, especially when they are alone. There are thousands of women who habitually have the smallest of appetites, and they are often enough women of a very active habit of body and brain. Want of appetite is much more common amongst women than amongst men, although it may be found in either sex.

We must distinguish between hunger and appetite. Hunger expresses a physical condition; appetite a mental condition. Sometimes we have an appetite, especially for some particular article of food, without being really hungry. Appetite is a stimulant to digestion; without it we are liable to digest badly. Sometimes it is not lack of appetite, but a feeling of not wanting to take the trouble to eat. There are many women who only like food which necessitates little effort to take and which by its qualities awakens to the least degree the psychic idea of eating; hence they eliminate most solid foods, which require a certain amount of chewing before they can be swallowed, and give preference to so-called light meals, which in some instances consist of no more than a cup of milk or cocoa and a couple of eggs. Sometimes the taking of food has been restricted with the idea of relieving some former digestive trouble. These are the patients who enter upon a strict regime which they follow only too well. By auto-observation and by auto-suggestion, by constantly noticing themselves and classifying their foods, and rejecting all kinds that they think they cannot digest, they finally manage to live on an incredibly small amount. Their attention may have been attracted to their digestion by some passing difficulty; such as the indigestion that all of us have at some time, and the idea that the stomach was not in order may have remained after the recovery; or they may have read or heard about certain articles of diet, and tabooed them. Whatever the origin, the effect of the attention paid to digestion is an anxiety at meals which prevents the relish of food, hinders the flow of the gastric juices, and thus interferes with proper assimilation. As long as the dyspepsia remains in the mind, just so long will the stomach continue to misbehave in sympathetic response to the mental state.

Many women say they have no appetite; that, even though they eat, their food has no taste. Such patients have lost their eating instinct to a certain degree. They eat merely from routine or because food is placed before them. They would usually just as soon not eat. If a number of courses be presented to them, they eat such as they care for and take a conventional amount of each kind of food presented; but they have no particular feeling to guide them in the matter of quantity. If they are in poor circumstances, and have not to prepare a meal for others, they are likely to neglect the preparation of one for themselves, to take almost anything that happens to be at hand, and then consider that they have eaten.

Now we all reason from our own experience far more than we do from what we obtain second-hand. And the familiar experience of everyone is that, when we have gone long without food, a stage is reached in which we do not care whether we have food or not; and it is easy under such circumstances to reject such food as is put into the stomach.

Another form of dyspepsia is due to failure of nervous power. A large number of dyspeptic women of the present day are so because their nervous power has diminished, or has been incontinently consumed in other directions without due regard for the needs of the stomach. Appetite is the best stimulant to digestion, but the patient who is fatigued has no appetite, therefore she digests badly. The act of taking food requires some effort, and effort is distasteful to these patients, especially when they have to order, or worse still, prepare their food. In some cases, indigestion is the first symptom of nervous exhaustion, and some time may elapse before other complaints are superadded. Its manifestations are almost endless. Loss or perversion of appetite, local discomfort or pain of various kinds and degrees, flatulent distension, eructations, nausea, and vomiting are the most prominent symptoms referable to the stomach. Often the patients feel worse when the stomach is empty, and are relieved by eating. In others, the symptoms appear after eating, though, perhaps, not until several hours have elapsed. The appetite is generally capricious. The capriciousness is sometimes so marked that the ingenuity of friends is severely taxed in the effort to provide sufficient nourishment for the patient. The symptoms not infrequently undergo a decided change for the better when the patient's mind is pleasantly occupied. Thus, when alone or with dull companions, food of any kind may be simply repulsive, and, if taken, may induce a host of painful sensations. But the same food, taken in the company of congenial associates, may be not only enjoyed by the palate, but digested with ease and comfort.

Another form of functional disorder of digestion arises from the variability of our moods. Worry and anxiety causes a condition of mental depression, the result being an impaired digestion and a lowered state of the nervous system. These women, as a result of their imperfect digestion, are almost always irritable, and find difficulty in exercising sufficient self-control to make life pleasant to themselves and their friends. People say that nothing affects the temper like disordered digestion, but the reverse is more correct; nothing troubles the functions of the stomach more than the mood we are in. People are not only sour in disposition because they are suffering from indigestion, but many are suffering from dyspepsia because they were previously out of sorts. All states of despondency disturb the process of digestion. They paralyse the secretory functions, and the muscular activities of both stomach and intestines. If the mind can be awakened and the spirits revived such patients will immediately begin to show improvement.

Disorders of the function of digestion are also common in hysterical subjects and assume various forms. The patients are wont to state that they feel, as it were, a ball rising from the pit of the stomach towards the throat, where it appears to remain, and causes a distressing sensation as if a foreign body were actually there, or as though the throat were compressed by a cord or by fingers. Some patients assert that they are unable to swallow, and this inability may continue until symptoms of inanition become prominent. Feelings of throat obstruction are common; so that patients not only refuse food, because, as they say, they cannot swallow, but also because the food seems to interfere with their breathing. The reasons given for not being able to swallow are numerous.

The stomach in these subjects is liable to show various indications of disorder. Obstinate longing for strange articles of food, loss of appetite, flatulence, pain, and vomiting, sometimes excessive, and continuing for lengthened periods, are among the most prominent of these symptoms. The vomiting occurs in severe cases every time food is taken, and the retching continues even when the stomach is completely emptied. Hysterical vomiting occurs during or immediately after meals; it is effortless and generally unaccompanied by nausea, so that the patient frequently feels ready to return to her meal immediately afterwards. The stomach is generally only partially emptied, so that nutrition is preserved; but in rare cases nothing is retained and severe emaciation results. When symptoms such as vomiting or abdominal pain occur in hysterical individuals, they may continue as the result of auto-suggestion after the original cause has disappeared.

In health there is a blessed unconsciousness of the very existence of a stomach, but let dyspepsia be present and the patient can think of little else. A healthy woman does not know that she has such a thing as a stomach, a dyspeptic woman does not know that she has anything else.

If there is merely a distaste for food it must be overcome by steady effort, taking definite quantities at regular intervals, whether wanted or not, whether liked or disliked, gradually adding to the amount. Appetite comes with eating. Without food there can be no permanent gain of strength; tonics cannot replace it, nor apothecary's potions be substituted for it, except for a short period in an emergency. Both stomach and bowels may be trained to perform their work regularly. Habit means probably more with them than any other factor. Our digestive tract is largely dependent on habit. If we accustom ourselves to dining every day at a particular hour, every day at that hour the stomach will become congested and secrete gastric juice without any intervention of our will. We get hungry three times a day or twice a day, according to the custom that we have established.

If there is real indigestion, that is another matter. But distaste for food, even discomfort in taking food, does not necessarily indicate indigestion. It may be merely that the stomach, long unused to the regular exercise of all its functions, is discontented at being asked to work, or is unready for work. All our organs form habits easily, the stomach most easily of any. If it is certain that only a rebellion is to be dealt with, it should be handled as in the former case by repeated and regular efforts to take food in moderate quantities without regard to the lack of desire for it.

In nervous patients with weak digestion, rest after meals is often beneficial. If digestion is only bad when the patient is fatigued, then a rest before meals is to be recommended. Patients with dainty or capricious appetites should not be discouraged by having too much food put before them or piling too much on their plates. They want to be coaxed by the daintiness with which their food is served. Another good rule for such patients is not to feed heavily at one meal, but to eat frequently a little and at regular intervals.

Many persons of middle age suffer through a monotony of diet. Our aim should be to keep our food range as wide as possible. Anything which tends to limit and monotonise diet exercises an injurious effect upon the general vigour of the system. Some people consume rather much of one article of diet. Generally speaking, men err as a rule in the excess of meat and alcohol, women in the excess of tea.

It is our duty to study the peculiarities and idiosyncrasies of the patient's stomach. Our stomachs are nearly as individual as our faces. But it is possible to go too far in humouring a capricious stomach. In persons of a nervous constitution, a too indulgent consideration for the care of this organ may entail disadvantages in regard to the general nutrition of the body, and produce effects which, in the long run, tend to lower the level of health, and even to aggravate that gastric sensitiveness which we are seeking to abate.

A woman who continuously and anxiously considers the kind of food she eats—whether it is going to agree with her or not—is a dyspeptic and will always remain so. The more completely she can keep her mind off her digestion and the "chemical" choice of her food, the better it is for her. It is not even always well for her to consider too nicely the amount of food taken or whether it is digestible or not. The really healthy stomach ought to be and is capable of disposing of not only the digestible and the difficult of digestion, but the indigestible. Any other kind of stomach is not worth having. At the same time, we must not forget that some perfectly wholesome foods are actual poisons to certain stomachs, and those which after repeated trials steadily disagree must be avoided. For food to be digested, it must first of all be agreeable to the taste. If it is agreeable, it will stimulate the juices indispensable to good digestion. Without appetite there is no healthy digestion, and food that palls on the appetite is just as surely non-effective as is food that is deficient in nutritive value. What is the use of telling the dyspeptic patient the nutritive properties of certain foods, if she cannot assimilate them? We must prescribe foods which the stomach will digest. All cases of nervous disorder want guidance and moral influence, more particularly in reference to diet than to any other curative agent; and each stomach must be treated according to its own respective requirements and, I might even go so far as to say, its own peculiarities.

Sometimes the patient's symptoms are so localised that they put one on the wrong scent, and the mistake is made of treating by local measures indigestion which originates in a disordered nervous system. No physician will neglect these local symptoms or fail to make a chemical examination; but in the class of patients of which this book treats the thoughtful physician will look upon the patient as a whole, not only from the point of view of the animal functions, but from the psychological point of view. He must consider not only what the patient eats or drinks, but be interested in what she thinks.

When the patient's indigestion is caused by the idea—not necessarily *conscious*—that she cannot digest, our treatment must be directed to the removal of the fixed idea. This is not always easy, for the patient is often sceptical from the frequent failures of the treatments she has already undergone; but I have seen patients whose dyspepsia has been treated for months by the ordinary methods who made a rapid recovery by the application of a suitable psychotherapy.

Let me add a few words about CONSTIPATION. Many more women are constipated habitually than men; there are many causes for it, but the commonest is physical inactivity. Another cause lies in the quantity and quality of food we eat. We take so much trouble nowadays to have it nourishing, digestible, and perfectly prepared that we often fail to give the stomach and intestines enough work to do. Another failing of women that brings about constipation is that of delaying to answer the calls of the system when they occur. Regularity in disposing of the waste products of the body is essential to healthy living. It is not only in the bad habits of the body, but in the bad habits of mind that the difficulty lies. Worry, nervousness, and low spirits delay and weaken the processes of digestion. Finally, there is the habit of taking laxatives, which, though they may help the patient out of a temporary inconvenience, do not remove the cause; and their constant use brings about a chronic condition, which the longer it lasts becomes the more difficult to treat. The majority of cases of constipation can be cured without drugs if proper treatment is instituted at a sufficiently early stage. In those cases in which purgatives must be used, an effort should be made to dispense with them at the earliest possible moment. Regular exercise in the open air is one of the most important means of prevention.

CHAPTER VII

NERVOUS DISORDERS OF THE HEART, CIRCULATION, AND RESPIRATION

THE circulation is often disturbed in nervous disorders. Sometimes there are palpitations and cardiac troubles, sometimes phenomena of vascular contraction (pallor) and vascular dilatation (blushing). The most frequent complaint is acceleration of the heart-beats, which is usually emotional in its origin. The moment the patient is approached, the pulse becomes rapid. Sometimes it is normal at the start, but accelerates from the time one begins to count it. A sudden noise, or a question which frightens the patient, is enough to make the heart gallop.

The heart has its own special work to do, and will do it well if left alone; but it represents a centre to receive and to distribute sympathy, through its nervous connections, greater than that of any other organ in the body. Everyone is only too familiar with the way in which the heart becomes affected by anything which disturbs the feelings, the emotions, and the sensitive nerve centres. It is influenced by every form of mental and moral emotion in a degree varying with the nervous state of the individual to whom it belongs, and it is also greatly influenced by the nature and character of the blood which circulates through it. Worry, suspense, anxious anticipation, disappointment, consciousness of failure or of failing health, the "hunted" feeling that comes of overwork and arrears, regret, sorrow, despair—all such depressing influences wear out not only the nervous system, with which they are immediately related, but the heart and blood-vessels as well.

There are unquestionably a larger number of women who are morbidly conscious of their heart's action. They feel disturbances, flutterings of the heart, throbbings, an intermission of their heart beating, or a faintness in its action. This condition, or group of conditions, is the result of purely nervous disorder. Many of these patients are in the habit of taking too little food; others hurry over their meals, eat too fast, or take tea to excess. Still others find their excitement in social entertainment.

Palpitation is a condition in which the patient is conscious of the beating of the heart; the severity varies from a mere sensation of fluttering to a violent and tumultuous throbbing and hammering of the heart against the chest wall during which the patient is in acute distress. These palpitations, and the distressing sensations by which they are accompanied, disturb the minds of the patients, who soon believe themselves to be affected with some grave lesion of the heart.

Besides the patients suffering from temporary palpitation, there are others, in whom the acceleration of the heart-beat is more permanent, owing to the mental condition being continually one of agitation. These patients are not overcome by any actual occurrence, but live in a continual state of uneasiness, in an agony of expectation, without being able to analyse their fears. This mental condition agitates the heart and gives rise to sensations which make the patient believe there is something organically wrong with the heart. It is not uncommon to hear a patient complaining of severe palpitations of the heart, worse at night when there is absolutely no exertion, and fearing heart disease when the heart is actually perfectly sound but the patient is suffering from anxious dreads of a definite or vague nature, which feeling of anxiety gives rise to unusual palpitation preventing sleep.

The pulsations of the nervous heart are distinctly felt by the patient as palpitations and have no gravity, but they return frequently, and their reappearance occurs under the influence of the most diverse and often the most trivial causes; a slight emotion, even a moderate physical effort, or the work of digestion, suffices to provoke them.

Sometimes the nervous heart is so irritable, so ill-tempered, so fractious, and so sensitive that it tumbles about, kicks, starts, and plunges in a manner which becomes exceedingly distressing and almost unbearable. At times the slightest movement of the body will produce this effect, walking upstairs, ascending a hill, reading a novel which touches the feelings, or the mere ordinary action of the bowels, or eating or drinking anything which disagrees. In this respect the heart is like the brain—a creature of habit. If one once lets it get out of training and assume vicious propensities, it takes a vast deal of moral persuasion, and something more, to put it right again.

Palpitations can, of course, arise from a variety of causes in perfectly healthy individuals, but they are not disturbed by them. It is our duty then to allay the fear of a patient. If the patient is at all sensible, this as a rule presents no difficulty. I have frequently brought down the heart-beats to their normal number by an appeal to the reason, somewhat as follows: The examination of the heart having revealed no abnormality, I tell the patient that her constitution is excellent; that she is in good health; that the palpitations of her heart are only nervous; that there are no symptoms of heart disease; that there is no danger whatever; that it is fear which throws her into the condition; that if she would lose the fear all her troubles would stop immediately; that if she can persuade herself that there is nothing the matter with herself she will lose her fears and her pulse will slow down, and that if she learns to repress by a healthy confidence in herself the timidity which makes her heart beat irregularly, she will keep her calmness of mind and her heart will stay quiet.

Having reassured the patient, the next point is to investigate the patient's mode of life. We may discover errors in the diet. Some are overworked. Others have little to do, but they are always in a hurry about it. Some patients, suffering from these functional derangements of the heart, make them a pretext for avoiding exercise and for taking stimulants, whereas exercise and fresh air are what they need.

Medicines in nervous affections of the heart

are generally useless. If there are some cases where they act favourably by suggestion, there are others, more numerous, where the use of an anodyne gives to the disease the stamp of reality, which is exactly what it ought not to have in the patient's mind. It awakens the idea of an organic affection, when the first consideration of the physician ought to be to dissipate all fear and all idea of danger.

GIDDINESS is another symptom which may occur in nervous women. The sensation is, as a rule, that of the early part of a fainting attack. Surrounding objects appear to be clouded and to be swaying, and the patient feels in need of steadying herself by holding on to something. Giddiness, however, may be more intense from a great variety of causes, organic as well as functional, and a correct diagnosis is of the first importance for successful treatment. Often the giddiness is merely an apprehension of giddiness, a fear of having an attack. When this dread seizes the patient she experiences a keen distress, and the state of confusion which accompanies the emotion is mistaken by her for an attack.

A form of ANGINA PECTORIS, a feeling of being gripped, a sensation of constriction of the chest with a feeling of terror, is not uncommon in nervous sufferers, but there is no organic lesion present. In functional angina pectoris, the main feature is sudden increase of blood pressure and a correspondingly sudden call upon cardiac effort. In these cases, whilst it is the heart that suffers the angina, the conditions which originate that suffering are outside the heart. It is none the less a source of anxiety for the persons attacked by it, and is peculiarly apt to throw them into a state of extreme dejection and depression.

Nervous angina comes on during repose, whereas the true form comes on after exertion. The attacks are often periodical and nocturnal, and may last an hour or two. It is as well that the patient should know that the attacks are never fatal; indeed, this pseudo-angina is quite compatible not only with continued good health, but with long life. Exaggeration of feeling due to concentration of attention plays a large rôle in these cases; and it is evident that the dread of something the matter with the heart, connected with even a slight sense of discomfort, may readily become so emphasised as to seem severe pain, though many people have similar feelings without making any complaint. For the treatment of this nervous form of angina, mental influence is all-important.

Nervous Disorders of the Circulation are extremely common in women. From the sympathetic system of nerves come the tiny nerve twigs—the vaso-motor nerves—which lie along the blood-vessels and regulate the circulation in the various parts of the body and limbs. When these little automatic regulators are weak and irritable, they are particularly susceptible to atmospheric conditions. Their possessor finds herself chilled and uncomfortable whenever the temperature, within doors and without, drops ever so slightly; and she finds that she cannot expose herself to the slightest draught of air without almost immediately experiencing the sensation of a cold in the head. Again, if the victim of vaso-motor irritability goes directly from an atmosphere in which she feels chilly into one which is at all hot, she finds herself, in a very short time, equally uncomfortable. Here, under the influence of the heat, the nerves in question allow too much blood to flow to the surface, with the result that the demand for an open window becomes imperative.

When these little nerves constrict the arteries, there is pallor and coldness of the body and a small pulse. These modifications are usually limited to the extremities of the limbs, producing the "dead fingers" sensation, and to the face.

They appear and disappear under the influence of various causes, such as an emotion, anxiety, or a sensation of cold. When the vascular spasm is general and sudden, it may cause intense and prolonged shivering, accompanied by trembling and a considerable fall of the peripheral temperature.

When these little nerves dilate the arteries there may be seen to appear blushes of redness disposed in patches over the face, chest, or extremities. This happens generally under the influence of excitation, and this dilatation of the vessels may alternate with states of constriction.

ABNORMAL PERSPIRATION is another symptom belonging to this category ; it is often associated with morbid blushing. The hands are the part usually affected, emotion or excitement causing a profuse perspiration to break out over the palms.

MORBID BLUSHING, although not strictly speaking a serious disorder, is, to say the least, extremely disagreeable to the victim. It is simply the manifestation of a weakness in the nervous system. It is not the symptom of blushing which needs treatment, but the general condition which is at the basis of the disorder. Probably the most prominent exciting cause is self-consciousness, either by introspection or by the attention being drawn to the external portions of the body while under observation by others.

Shy and nervous persons blush readily when attention or remarks are directed to their personal appearance. If a modest young woman of a delicate nervous organisation is in company with a number of persons and imagines that the people around her are regarding her critically, she is very liable to manifest her abnormal self-consciousness by blushing, or even by becoming embarrassed in her conversation, and stammering.

Blushing is generally confined to the face, on account of its extreme vascularity, and therefore, having a greater supply of vaso-motor nerves, emotional disturbances manifest themselves more prominently in that part, the face being the portion of the body most exposed to view and upon which most attention is concentrated in looking for recognition, or in studying character or discerning beauty and comeliness. When the blushing is of a severe type there is always mental confusion present. In a large number of cases the individual completely loses the power of thought for the time being. The mind is paralysed, and, in popular language, she is " covered with confusion." There is an instinctive desire for self-concealment. The blusher either averts the head or looks with downcast eyes. The expression " I wished I could have sunk through the floor " aptly expresses the mental condition of the patient. The blush is often followed by pallor of the face; this is due, as before explained, to constriction of the blood-vessels—a reaction following their dilatation.

Morbid blushing occurs frequently in women exhausted by anxiety and overwork. When a person has once suffered from this disorder she is liable to have recurrent attacks, as the nervous system is highly impressionable, and the condition once well developed is apt to be perpetuated by slight influences, such as disordered digestion. The flushed cheeks and red nose due to this nervous disorder are a source of great mortification and mental distress to those so affected. It is a most disagreeable affliction to women. Such persons are frequently condemned as secret drinkers when perhaps there is nothing wrong with them other than a slight gastric catarrh.

This complaint is of course most serious to teachers, artists, and other professional women who have to earn their living. The treatment has to be directed to the removal of the cause, the exaggerated self-consciousness. By suggestion treatment we can inspire the patient with more self-esteem and teach her to regard the presence of others with more or less indifference. Any physical defect or disorder must of course be attended to as well.

Nervous disorders of respiration are often noticed in nervous women; for instance, slight acceleration of the respiratory movement, irregularities of rhythm, and sighs. Many complain of a purely subjective sensation of distress. Shortness of breath is often a trying symptom, especially for stout people, and prevents them from taking necessary exercise. When it cannot be traced directly to some affection of the heart or of the circulatory apparatus, it is usually due to lack of exercise. Much can be done for it by deliberate training. Anyone who has seen the shallow breathing of many of the patients who go to Nauheim, and how much it has improved by the gradually increased walks up the hills around the valley, will appreciate how much training in deep breathing means.

Loss of voice is another symptom often dependent upon psychic causes in women whose profession depends on the exercise of their vocal cords. On examination no abnormal physical signs can be found, and the aphonia only occurs at irregular intervals, commences suddenly, and passes away rapidly. If the history of the patient be minutely examined, it will in all probability transpire that there has been some slight and unimportant organic affection; this was accompanied by worry due to the inability of the patient to carry on her work, and, though of itself of small moment, apprehension of a recurrence has remained and shows itself at times in specimens of what would happen if, in fact, the affection were to return. In the case of a patient whose malady is of the larynx or of the respiratory passages in general, the association of troubles of these regions with the idea of cold being very common, it is quite likely that fussy precautions against the supposed effects of cold will be much in evidence. Among such persons, we find those who shelter themselves from cold to such a degree that life becomes one round of searching for and avoiding possible draughts, or of varying the number of layers of their clothing with the level of the thermometer.

Spasm of the larynx is a peculiar nervous symptom. There are few of us who, at some time of our lives, have not known the sensation of choking in the throat from emotion. It is a brief and unpleasant experience, and for healthy people an uncommon one; but among highly nervous people there is a rare form of this trouble which gives rise to temporary loss or inhibition of voice. At first from emotion, worries, or without known cause, there is felt in or about the larynx a sense of momentary strangling and pain. If the person is speaking the voice breaks and she becomes speechless, or the voice becomes shrill and then breaks. At every effort there is pain, distress referred to the larynx, and squeaky, broken tones. There is also a sense of constriction, and sometimes the œsophagus seems to share in the annoyance, and an upward gulping effort follows or accompanies the laryngeal disturbance.

I saw some years ago a well-educated girl, twenty years of age, who originally suffered from a choking sensation in her throat with a feeling of anxious depression. Subsequently she happened one day to take a piece of meat in her mouth of rather larger size, which actually obstructed her air passage so that she was nearly suffocating, but after an attack of coughing she succeeded in emitting it again. Instead of realising that she ought to have cut her food more finely and masticated it properly, she, from that time, formed the delusion that she was unable to swallow solids because of a constriction in her throat, i.e. of her œsophagus. She would only take liquid foods, and as that was insufficient, she rapidly lost weight. She made a perfect recovery by " suggestion " treatment.

Asthma. There is a form of asthma—a spasm of the bronchial tubes—common to nervous women, which is often precipitated directly by the influence of the emotional and imaginative faculties: by anger, joy, fear, or by the outbreak of a thunderstorm, or by being left alone in the dark. Other causes are: irritation set up by dust, fog, pollen, scent, and even of cold air. Irritation in almost any part of the body may lead to a paroxysm. Sometimes the attacks are limited to certain localities: at a certain elevation, or on the sea level, or actually at sea. The point to be remembered is that they occur in patients psychically predisposed to them.

Spasmodic asthma is not an incurable disease, but is in most cases amenable to rational treatment by eliminating the exciting causes, and treating by suggestion the underlying and ever-present psychical factor.

CHAPTER VIII

LOSS OF MUSCULAR CONTROL
NERVOUS TREMORS AND MUSCULAR SPASMS

Nervous Tremors, besides being an expression of weakness, as in old age, fatigue, the feebleness of convalescence, organic disease, or toxic states, are in many people a sign of transient emotion, of fear, excitement, anger, or of grief, almost as natural in some mobile natures as laughter or crying is of uncontrolled mirth or grief. In some persons almost any position or action in which they feel themselves under observation causes a tremor. Such tremor is capable in nervous persons of passing over the line of healthy functional manifestation. It commonly ceases during rest. It is often controlled for a time, but no less often, it is made worse by the determined effort of the patient to overcome the affection, making her more conscious of it than before; and by the fear of trembling, and the discomfort which it causes, reacting on the emotional state, which makes the trembling lasting. The parts affected are chiefly the hands and the head.

Persons affected with tremors always complain more of this symptom when they are in a run-down condition; therefore in treating this complaint we must attend to the general health, besides giving such "suggestion" treatment as will train the patient to secure psychic control over herself and her muscles.

Nervous Tics are muscular spasms due to hypersensitiveness of the nervous system. The movement, which constitutes the tic, originally served a definite purpose, but has become exaggerated and can be controlled only, if at all, at the cost of great mental discomfort. The patient realises the foolishness of her tic, and a conflict occurs between the illogical desire to perform it and the logical desire to restrain it. The exciting causes of tic are the same as those of general nervous exhaustion, namely, emotional excitement, mental and physical shock, strain, and any condition which lowers the general health.

In simple tics the facial muscles are most often affected, but the head, shoulder, or arms may also be involved, and sniffing or coughing and every variety of weird sound may occur. Often it is originally merely a response to some irritation, as for instance when the eye is screwed up in the effort to see with an uncorrected error of refraction. This motor response is normal, but it becomes abnormal when it continues after its cause has disappeared, as it then no longer serves any useful purpose. An occasional blink is thus replaced by a series of futile flickerings of the eyelids. It is seldom that more than one tic is practised at a time. Some special kind of grimace may persist for days or weeks, and then cease as suddenly as it began, only to give place to other forms of tic in succession. The tic becomes most evident upon excitement or fatigue, and increases with self-consciousness. The patients sometimes imagine that they can repress their movements, but this is, as a rule, wasted effort. The attention of the patient is thereby fastened on the tic and on the sensations and ideas which have caused it, and the impulsion becomes still more irresistible.

Although such patients may be, and often are, of high intelligence and fertile in imagination, they usually present on careful investigation definite evidence of mental instability and eccentricities. They are often irresolute, lacking in perseverance, and are subject to vagary and caprice. Tics are also not infrequently associated with obsessions and with various phobias, such as fear of open or enclosed spaces. Indeed the recognition of the mental condition is a fact of the first practical importance. The whole treatment of tic depends upon it. It should, in short, have a double object: the correction of the unreasonable motor manifestation by removal of the irritating cause, and the correction of the psychic anomalies. It is best not to notice the movements of these patients, not to speak of them either, but to calm the primary emotion, the fear of the spasm. Everything must be done to interest them in other directions and make them forget their trouble, to overcome their timidity and self-consciousness. We must explain to them the effects of fear and expectant attention, and get them to regard their spasmodic movements with indifference. In this manner, even if they are not stopped at once, they can be lessened in intensity and frequency, and through this means the patient will be encouraged and gradually acquire complete control.

Writers' Cramp is one of the most common examples of *occupation neuroses*. These affections present one feature which is common to them all, namely, that certain actions, previously accomplished with perfect ease, are rendered difficult or even impossible in consequence of cramp, tremor, paralysis, or acute neuralgic pain, whereas other movements are performed by the same muscles without difficulty or discomfort. As a matter of course the upper extremity, and particularly the hands and fingers, are most liable to be thus affected, inasmuch as these parts have more work thrown on them. Whatever lowers the general tone of the nervous system may act as a predisposing cause, but the most usual cause met with is anxiety due to family trouble, business worry, or weighty responsibilities in persons whose avocations require them to write for many hours daily. The mental element in these cases is shown by the frequency with which the intensity of the cramp corresponds to the amount of attention which is directed to the act. The majority of the sufferers are those who are compelled to write a good legible hand and overtax their muscles. The chief disturbance is usually from spasm, but sometimes it is from pain. The spasm may be limited to the act of writing, and other actions, such as piano-playing or painting, may be performed without the slightest difficulty. It is a troublesome and difficult affection to treat; but by attention to the cause and by electrical treatment, which must be adapted to each case, cures are often achieved. What has been said of tics is true to some extent of writers' cramp; and where the mental condition is at fault, judicious psychotherapeutic methods must be applied. The introduction of typewriting has largely diminished the number of patients suffering from this complaint.

PIANOFORTE-PLAYERS' CRAMP is a similar affection occurring chiefly amongst professional pianists. Seeing the possibility of being forced to abandon their art, which may be the sole means of their livelihood, they become profoundly depressed and their anxiety still further aggravates their complaint.

CHOREA, or the disease commonly known as St. Vitus's dance, is a nervous affection which most frequently occurs in childhood, is quite often met with in young women, and is found sometimes during pregnancy. Rarely also it may manifest itself at the change of life. The exciting cause may be a fright, or any violent disturbance of the emotions. It is in children often associated with rheumatism. This disorder is characterised by irregular spasmodic movements, by inco-ordination of voluntary movement, and often by muscular and mental weakness and irritability of temper. The first thing to attract attention is sometimes the spontaneous twitching in the hands or face. Objects which are being carried are suddenly dropped. The spasmodic movements are occasional only, but their frequency increases with their severity, until at last they may be so continuous and violent that the limbs are in constant agitation. The movements are unilateral, the left being the side most frequently affected, and they are always increased by excitement and by attempts at voluntary movement, and almost invariably cease during sleep.

As regards treatment, hygienic rest is needed, long hours of sleep, a period of lying down in the afternoon; but above all such occupation of mind with simple, pleasant, yet interesting things, needing not much exercise, as will keep their attention from themselves. There is nothing like "suggestion" treatment for these cases.

Chronic Spasms occur in hysterical women and may involve almost any part of the body. The jaw may be locked, the head may be bent on the breast, and the legs drawn up, and the contracted muscles may be held in that position for months.

Catalepsy is a condition akin to chronic spasm and occurs likewise in hysterical girls. The limbs may remain in an awkward wax-like state. Some time ago I had a patient, a well-developed country girl, nineteen years of age, who suffered from these attacks. For example, while dressing herself and tying a knot with the strings of her petticoat she would suddenly stop still like a wax figure, all muscles becoming rigid. If her mother tried to move a limb she would experience a slight resistance, but the limb would continue in the new position just as rigid. Calling to her would not rouse her, although the girl recollected everything that happened when she came to.

Other Spasms that occur in nervous subjects are spasms of the internal muscles. Thus the lump in the throat, or "globus," is very common, vomiting through spasm of the stomach, difficulty in swallowing through spasm of the œsophagus leading to great wasting from want of solid food, bronchial spasms leading to attacks of asthma, and lastly spasms of limbs and groups of muscles, simulating in its worst form, when accompanied by convulsions, an epileptic attack.

Genuine Epilepsy, or the falling sickness, is really an organic disease, though its pathology is still unknown. It may be mentioned here, however, that attacks are sometimes brought on from emotional causes, such as worry, anxiety, and especially fright. It is characterised by sudden attacks of unconsciousness, which may or may not be followed by convulsions. The majority of epileptics date their affliction from early life, and in a number of women it is closely allied to migraine. Occasionally the two diseases may alternate or coincide in the same patient. The frequency of the attacks may range from one or two in a lifetime to several in a day. The fits are generally more numerous about the time of the menstrual period, and in some occur only at night. The fit may or may not be preceded by an *aura*, a sensation such as a rising from the pit of the stomach into the chest and throat, or giddiness, tingling in the limbs, or a sensation of a peculiar smell, lasting a few seconds. The patient gets rigid all over, head and eyes may turn to one side, the colour of the face becomes dusky, and this is followed by repeated jerking contractions of the whole body. The tongue may be bitten in the contraction of the jaws. When the convulsions have ceased the patient lies flaccid, breathing stertorously, and may either regain consciousness rapidly or may lie in a deep sleep for some hours. In those in whom fits are frequent, signs of mental deterioration are common.

Hystero-Epilepsy is a term applied to

designate severe convulsive attacks exactly similar to the paroxysms of true epilepsy, but occurring in hysterical subjects and being a purely functional disorder. These attacks can be distinguished from genuine epilepsy by the fact that hysterical patients do not hurt themselves when throwing themselves about, taking care where they propose to fall; whereas the epileptic is so completely unconscious that she has no choice. In the delirium of hystero-epilepsy the patients are vociferous, singing, dancing, and being at one moment difficult to restrain, while immediately after, they are sunk in deep confusion.

MINOR EPILEPSY OR PETIT MAL is a form of epilepsy in which there is loss of consciousness without convulsions. The patient suddenly stops in her occupation, looks strange for a moment, and then goes on with what she is doing; may even finish a sentence she had commenced, and be aware of what has happened only by finding that she has dropped something which was in her hands, or that she is the object of anxious observation. In some patients the loss of consciousness is preceded by some warning sensation, and it is from this circumstance that these seizures are so often termed "sensations." The patient may know nothing of the loss of consciousness, and be aware only of the preliminary sensation. Others who are ignorant of the seriousness of their complaint describe their attacks simply as "faints," "turns," or "giddiness." After the attack is over the patient may be at once quite well; but more often she is stupid and dull for a time, and in some cases she proceeds to perform some action in a dream-like, automatic manner, such as undressing herself, retaining afterwards no recollection of what she has done.

Larvated Epilepsy. In this form of epilepsy the attacks are usually very infrequent and may be altogether overlooked, though the period of automatism that follows may be prolonged for hours or days, or even longer. These attacks are generally known as loss of memory. Suddenly, without warning, the patient passes into a subconscious state and may disappear from her friends, turning up perhaps days afterwards many miles from home. In this state she may wander about or travel by train and behave sufficiently naturally not to attract attention.

As regards the causes and pathology of epilepsy there is still considerable difference of opinion. Sometimes "Bromide" treatment effects a cure. The patient should avoid anything that irritates the nervous system, anything that exhausts the nervous energy, anything that disturbs the emotional balance, and should beware of indigestion and constipation, as these are the forerunners of epileptic attacks in the vast majority of instances. I have applied "suggestion" treatment with gratifying results in a number of cases, where objection was taken to medicinal remedies. Certainly for hystero-epilepsy there is no better treatment.

CHAPTER IX

EMOTIONAL INSTABILITY

HYSTERIA

WOMEN suffering from disordered nerves usually show a loss of control over their emotions, which thus become too active. They become capricious, unreasonable, selfish, and react easily to slight causes. Thus at times they are gay, active, and mischievous; at other times, dreamy, passive, and apathetic to their surroundings, or extremely irritable. Laughter and crying are repressed with difficulty, and recur on the slightest provocation. A chance word or some trivial action, without any malicious intent on the part of someone present, is sufficient to elicit the kaleidoscopic change. As a rule, these emotional manifestations are aroused by the patient being thwarted in doing something she wished to do, or in being compelled to do something she did not wish to do. Such persons have little power of self-control; they torture themselves and others with their morbid nervousness, and though frequently quick in repartee and conversation of a superficial kind, are lacking in judgment and incapable of carrying out any intricate or extended study to a definite end. When married they are the terror of husbands, who find all plans of conduct towards their wives a failure; for hardly has the husband determined on one line of conduct, than he finds his wife changed again. In their love affairs they must have romance; and if they are not themselves sought after, they seek to interfere with the love affairs of others. False accusations of a sexual nature are common with them. All is caprice with them. They love without measure those whom they will soon hate without reason. Their needs are constantly changing. They are extravagantly affectionate, or callous and indifferent by turns; selfish, clamouring for sympathy, aggrieved and infuriated by any thwarting of their immediate desires; enthusiastic and overjoyed or needlessly depressed and abased by inadequate causes; arrogant, boastful, and apparently determined one day, and the next timid, self-depreciatory, and irresolute. They are the prey of every passing fancy or mood, and soon become exhausted by emotional excesses; yet unless supplied with a daily changing menu of stirring feelings they speedily become bored, introspective, and hypochondriacal. This emotional instability varies of course in degree, and is rare among women who have serious interests in life.

Intellectually they are often above the average, quick at learning though forgetful, seldom capable of prolonged industry, but working with feverish energy in fits and starts. In conversation they exaggerate everything with tiresome reiteration. The superlative degree is called into use at every turn. A large number are given to lying and slandering, and stories of the most extraordinary character may be invented by these patients. They have little power of application, as a rule, and are always talking of how tired and weak they are; yet they will spend hours in pottering about, and give infinite thought and time to trifles that ought to be disposed of summarily. Whims of the most varied kind are invented from time to time; those who point out their absurdity are regarded as enemies. They have been known to starve themselves, to refuse to walk or to speak for years, to mutilate themselves, even torture themselves, in order to produce strange and puzzling symptoms. They not only imagine themselves the victims of the most diverse and serious diseases, but by some obscure power, they unconsciously simulate diseases, of the symptoms of which they themselves cannot possibly have any knowledge. The whole household is kept busy ministering to their slightest feeling of discomfort, which is dwelt upon and exaggerated till the patient grows to believe herself to be suffering cruelly. Everybody and everything must bend to their feelings and their views. Their obstinacy is extreme, and their regard for the point of view of others is entirely swallowed up in their own way of looking at a given thing and dealing with it.

The world is full of these unstable, sensitive and emotional women. Suggestibility is their dominant quality, or, more exactly, auto-suggestibility.

One characteristic of these patients is that their attention soon wearies and they become absent-minded; they dream; they abstract themselves, so to speak, from their surroundings; they become self-hypnotised.

The dreamy states that are experienced in some of these cases may be of short or long duration. Sometimes the patients go about in these dream-states, performing various acts with little or no recollection of them on returning to consciousness. In other cases, they claim to have seen visions, to have heard beatific music, or to have undergone most frightful experiences, regardless of all efforts of the bystanders to "bring them to their senses." Some grow extremely fantastic or silly, or sentimental in behaviour, laugh immoderately, cry uproariously, scream, sing, or shout unreasonably.

In some cases these patients are subject to a mild form of delirium. The mildest type consists simply of talking during sleep; but in the more severe forms, the patient leaves the bed and walks about, and if the excitement be still more marked she may even go into the street and walk long distances. Upon waking in the morning, there may be a faint recollection of what has occurred, as *somnambulism*—as the disease is called—is really only a very pronounced form of dreaming of which movement forms a part.

Again, in some of these patients, as the result of a series of acute attacks, the patient may lose the remembrance of all the past events of her life, and only recollect them during a subsequent attack. These are described as cases of *double personality*. Such patients seem possessed of two or more personalities, so that in one state they seem conscious of certain experiences, and live up to a certain character, while in another state they seem entirely different beings. In each state they remember only the events of the life which correspond to such state, and forget those of the other.

Derangement of sensibility is a very common nervous disorder in these women. There may be anæsthesia, i.e. loss of sensibility, affecting usually the skin only, but sometimes also the deeper structures, and occurring either in patches or extending to one half of the body, generally the left side; or, what is more frequently the case, there may be hyperæsthesia, over-sensitive spots on various parts of the body. Sometimes the whole cutaneous surface is more sensitive than usual. Tingling and numbness in the extremities may occur and at times the sensory irritability may become so pronounced that sharp, darting pains of a neuralgic character may appear.

Often there is a general loss of muscular power, leading to *hysterical paralysis*. The simple belief that a muscle cannot be contracted or relaxed, the conviction of her helplessness, is sufficient in such a patient to render the muscles immovable. It is the mental state of the patient —an error in mental representation—which is responsible, in a great measure, for her inability to initiate movements. The paralysis may comprise a single limb or an entire side of the body, or it may be limited to one muscle of the eye, or to the vocal cords. When the eye muscles are involved the patient sees images double; when the vocal cords are involved, there is produced an hysterical loss of voice known as aphonia. One of the most frequent forms of hysterical paralysis is that in which the patient is unable to walk, although the limbs may be freely used and moved when the patient is lying down. Sometimes a limb is not actually paralysed and yet there may be an inability to move the limb, due to muscular contracture following the pain of a slight injury, after which the patient feels unable to move the limb and finally becomes possessed with a fixed idea that all active or spontaneous movements are impossible. These hysterical paralyses only outwardly resemble the real organic paralyses of the nervous system. Apart from other distinctions, there is one important one: no matter how long the paralysis may persist, no wasting of the paralysed muscles follows, such as would take place in an organic paralysis.

Sometimes there is a spasmodic contraction of muscles, especially the neck muscles, twisting the head or bending the head from the left or right, producing what is known as hysterical wry-neck. Occasionally the muscular spasm involves the diaphragm and produces disturbances of respiration or persistent hiccough.

Heredity is the great predisposing factor in hysteria, the disease occurring particularly in the offspring of neuropathic parents. Emotions of various sorts, particularly fright and terror, or the suppression of painful experiences are among the chief direct provoking agents. Fatigue may also be a factor. But it is the disposition to mental abstraction, to absent-mindedness, which accounts for the various subconscious phenomena. The mind is too narrow to take in a number of ideas at the same time, and certain perceptions do not enter consciousness; in other words, there is a retraction of the field of consciousness. In anæsthesia, it is sensation which escapes personal perception; in paralysis, it is movement; in loss of memory or amnesia, the storing up or conservation of impressions is entirely disregarded by the patient and hence reproduction of these impressions is at fault. The retraction of the field of consciousness either gives too much power to certain ideas or causes certain ideas temporarily to drop out of the field of conscious perception.

The increased suggestibility accounts also for the long line of symptoms.

There is no one line of treatment for the

disease. The treatment must be modified according to the cause of the disease, its evolution, its particular symptoms, by the social condition and age of the patient, and finally by the patient's personality. It consists both of physical and moral therapy. The patient is best separated from her home surroundings, which are often full of discord and harmful suggestions, and placed under the care of trained and kind nurses. The general health must be attended to; hyper-alimentation on Weir Mitchell lines does good; and the individual symptoms such as the paralysis, anæsthesia, convulsions, contractures, pains, tremors, will require appropriate treatment, such as electricity and massage. The tendency to increased suggestibility and emotionalism must be combated. Re-education of the emotions is of great importance; but whether this re-education should be accomplished by isolation, persuasion, suggestion, the personality of the physician, psycho-analysis, or by ignoring the symptoms, is a matter of individual technique, so long as we aim at the acquisition of self-control, the proper direction of the Will, and stop the patient from indulging in her morbid imagination and reverie. Diversion of mind is also important. Many of these patients, as I have pointed out repeatedly, have either no serious interests with which to occupy themselves, or their interests are not engrossing and can be put off whenever they wish. Duties that are inevitable, and that call for the occupation of so much time that the patient has little opportunity to think of herself, are often the salvation of these women.

MENSTRUATION. It is well known that in diseases of the womb and ovaries, nervous and mental disturbances are common; but even with apparently healthy organs, the functions peculiar to women influence the mental state. Menstruation is, of all the functions of the feminine organisation, that which acts the most on the brain and nervous system. There is in many women either an exaltation with excitation of the mental functions, or a corresponding lowering and depression of these. During these periods of excitation or depression women, who at other times are in every respect normal in their acts and social relationships, manifest abnormalities in their characters and in their mental attitudes. Practically all the peculiarities of the individual are emphasised at these times, and if there are any special neurotic conditions or psychic anomalies, they become quite marked. A woman under the influence of her periods becomes more easily tired and more sensitive, more emotional, and more a prey to her auto-suggestions, than when in her normal condition. Her tears flow more readily, she is less able to bear annoyances. She gets fretful, peevish, capricious, and bad-tempered. Sometimes the influence is shown by the brain feeling muddled, by failing memory, and distressing headaches. One often finds in her a spirit of contradiction which she does not show at any time except during the menstrual period. Irritability is common. Many a domestic misunderstanding begins at these times and is unfortunately allowed to continue because the real reason for it—the instability of disposition due to menstruation—is not recognised. Often affections that are always present give symptoms only during the menstrual period or just before it. The more claims a woman has on her attention, the less likely is she to be bothered at the monthly periods; indeed, the majority of women pass through it absolutely undisturbed.

The nutritional disturbances to which all women are subjected during PREGNANCY allow few of them to escape, at least, some alteration of the disposition. When slight, these changes are manifested principally in the form of capriciousness, abnormal appetites and cravings, tendencies toward brooding over possible ill results of the pregnancy to themselves, or some slight degree of mental exaltation, in which the imagination is more particularly disturbed. In severer cases, there may be a special dislike and distrust of the husband, and aversion from the children. In their antipathy toward the husband, these women imagine that their husbands do not love and sympathise with them as they should. Some careless word or sentence spoken in merriment may be interpreted as evidence that their friends no longer care for them, especially if they have failed to visit them as often as formerly. They are confident that other women have never suffered as they are suffering, and they may experience imperfectly defined apprehensions of approaching danger. In a number of cases, they suspect their husband of infidelity, fancy that they are going to be abandoned, or that their children are to be taken from them. There may be complete apathy and loss of interest in family and surroundings, and weariness of life.

Pregnant women in the more advanced state experience longings for various things, chiefly for articles of diet. Sometimes, however, the longing extends to articles of dress, or jewels, and becomes irresistible; and a theft may be committed. Such kleptomania can be distinguished from ordinary thieving by various considerations. The patient may be rich and by no means ungenerous with her money; the article appropriated may be comparatively worthless or of no practical value to her; or if of value, it may not be appreciated once it is taken and may be put away or replaced.

During the first few weeks *after delivery of the child*, there may be again mental and nervous disturbances in those predisposed to it. *Prolonged feeding of the infant* may also cause exhaustion and anæmia, and affect the mental and physical health of the mother.

The *Change of Life* in women often produces serious nervous disturbances and mental changes of so varied a character, that we have devoted a special chapter to it.

CHAPTER X

THE CHANGE OF LIFE

A CRITICAL period as regards nervous disorders is what has been aptly described as the autumn time of a woman's life. Her spring and summer have gone by. As in the plant when flower- and seed-time have passed, so is she entering on that which produces the "fall," that which ushers in the winter of old age. Nature is kind to the majority of women and imperceptibly prepares the system for the change, so that the crisis is passed through with comparatively little trouble. In some, on the other hand, the event affects profoundly the entire organisation, mental and physical. It is a real "change of life" with them.

The change of life not only terminates critically many complaints of the preceding years, but it governs the state of health during the whole subsequent period of life; so much so that, from the manner in which this crisis is accomplished, it is possible to predict whether, in after-life, health will be good or bad. That women often gain additional strength of constitution is shown by the greater longevity of women, by their being less liable to sudden death, and by their general immunity from disease. This invigoration of health is sometimes accompanied by a very great improvement of personal appearance, when the emaciated put on a fair amount of fat, which is both comely and conducive to health. Many women, like roses, retain their sweetness long after they have lost their beauty; while others do not recover health without some sacrifice of feminine grace, their appearance becoming more masculine, the bones projecting more than previously, while the skin is less unctuous, and stray hairs may appear on the face.

Women who have led well-regulated lives, and have been healthy and free from worries of mind and strain of body before the change, may escape from many of the minor ailments which are so very usual at this time. Thankful that they have escaped from real sufferings, women cease to torture themselves with imaginary woes; and as they feel the ground grow steadier underfoot they are less dependent on others, and often at the evening of life they derive happiness from an increased disposition to religion, charity, friendship, and material affection.

The revolution effected throughout the whole system by the cessation of sexual life often causes indirectly mental changes of less pleasant a nature. When the hereditary and personal history has been good, and there has been no special stress, the change takes place so gradually as to be imperceptible. All the mental powers are lessened in activity to a certain degree, and the woman has to adapt herself to their reduced energies. She realises that she has arrived at a great epoch of existence ; not only does she feel the approach of old age with its attendant infirmities, but she knows that she is about to lose the peculiar characteristic of her sex.

Life's enjoyment has diminished and fatigue sets in more readily. At the same time, the defence against disease is lowered, and often this is the beginning of the end, the time when the first signs of that illness appear, to which, in after years, the individual succumbs. For both sexes, the climacterium is a period for the re-adaptation of the bodily machinery to a more modified functional activity. If, then, there are cares and sorrows, mental or physical over-exertion, it will be more difficult than ever to retain the normal elasticity. At any other time the body would have recovered easily. Now there is not enough vitality and nervous energy, or only after a period of long inactivity.

The tired condition often implies an instinctive feeling that work, exertion, and effort are not always entirely worth while. Physiologically and psychologically, energising by itself is no longer felt to be so necessary. The tired feeling often leads to a lowering in the desires and ideals. Pleasures that cost little and imply small exertion are preferred to pleasures of the higher sort that need some strenuousness to attain them. Many women take to alcohol, then, because it seems to them to be the simplest way of reviving some of the intensities of their former lives or of deadening their regrets, and over-indulgence is common.

In some women at this period there are apt to arise what may be called obsessional feelings —that is, strange ideas come into the mind against their will and in a dominant and irresistible way. They come like strangers unbidden to a feast. Such ideas may be merely theoretical, in other cases they tend towards some kind of action of an unreasonable kind. A woman takes it into her mind that she had neglected some duty in regard to a dead child, or that her thoughts had wandered to improper subjects during her prayers, or that she had not educated her children in the right way; or she gets the impression that she has some incurable disease of a certain organ, generally cancer, and is quite incredulous when assured that the particular organ is healthy. Many women become difficult to please and sharp-spoken, irritability of temper is common; and perhaps it is to this reason, in part, that one must attribute the proverbial bad reputation which in every country is given to a great many mothers-in-law.

Like the flickering flame before it extinguishes will often burn up higher and brighter, so the sexual instinct before it is lost will show abnormal functioning; and many a woman at this "dangerous age" will do "silly" things, fall in love with a much younger man, who spurns her, and conduct herself in a manner that makes her the laughing-stock of her friends. Erotic delusions may occur. The revival of the passion may cause the wife to believe that she is neglected for some other woman, or a feeling of antipathy to the husband may arise which becomes misinterpreted for dislike on his part. In either case, the woman becomes suspicious and is on the look-out for evidence, when trifles, light as air, suffice to satisfy her. One woman searches her husband's pockets, while another deciphers in a mirror the writing on his blotting-pad.

When once the false idea has become established, reason is of no avail. During this stage of insane jealousy acts of violence and destructiveness are common, and frequently injurious letters and post cards are written, thus causing general scandal.

I have known many women at the climacteric take most preposterous and obsessional notions as to gentlemen paying attention to them and proposing marriage. If such an idea remains a mere thought, kept to herself or merely communicated to her intimate friends, it is all very well; but I have known it result in very unpleasant persecution of the supposed lovers and in most ludicrous acts with serious consequences. After having lived in a most exemplary manner up to the change of life, some women have deserted husband and children for a scamp; while others only stay at home, to make it intolerable by their tyrannical conduct, and hate the long-cherished objects of their former affection.

Often the changes are so slight that they are not noticed by relatives and friends in the daily domestic life of the woman, but sometimes the changes amount almost to insanity. Thus an expression of physical and mental inaptness and fatigue in a previously active-minded and energetic woman ; an unusual excitability and irritability in one hitherto of an even and placid disposition ; an obvious loss of interest in amusements, social pursuits, and domestic occupations, which before had given pleasure ; a proneness to constant complaints of pains, which are not justified by any local condition, in one who had usually been uncomplaining and self-restraining ; the unexplained and sudden dislikes to friends and even near relatives, where before there had been friendly and affectionate relationships ; a brooding over trifles, depressing anticipations and apprehensions of imaginary losses, appearing in a temperament which had always been hopeful and bright ; these are the graver symptoms of the psychic changes occasionally produced. If such is the case, the woman requires judicious management and constant watchfulness, and the presence of a nurse who is familiar with the management of this class of patient.

Like the mental symptoms, so the physical signs are of great variety.

In some there is persistent insomnia, while in others—women who have suffered from profuse blood losses—there is drowsiness due to anæmia of the brain.

Another common complaint is irregularity of

the heart. The patient suffers from severe palpitations, from difficulty of breathing after exertion, from cardiac distress, faintness, and rapid pulse. Throbbing of the vessels of the head and neck, pricking sensations in the limbs, coldness of the extremities, etc., are very frequently experienced. The symptoms may constitute definitely recurring attacks, and may make the patient think she has heart disease.

At the change of life most women have the power of generating a more than usual amount of heat ; they often want less clothing, and even in winter leave their doors and windows wide open. Very often, however, instead of being regularly distributed, this heat bursts forth as flushes, women feel as if something started from the pit of the stomach, spreading over the chest, and then over the face, which becomes suffused and hot. I have heard women compare their sensations to burning steam rising from the middle of the body to the head. These flushes may follow or precede a chill, or a momentary sensation of shivering or sinking and faintness. If the flushes do not terminate in a gentle moisture of the skin, women call them "dry heats." The face and chest generally suffer most from flushes, but the whole of the skin may be affected, and the hands and nails may feel like fire.

There may be dyspepsia, generally of a functional kind, as well as so-called bilious attacks.

Headache is a very usual symptom at the change of life. Many patients complain that, since the periods became irregular or ceased, they suffer from violent headaches, either in the temples, the top of the head, across the forehead, or less frequently in the back of the head.

There may be defects of vision, and there may be varying degrees of weakness of the intrinsic muscles of the larynx with alterations in the voice. The auditory apparatus may be affected, with a resulting hypersensitiveness and intolerance of certain sounds, and diverse forms of noises in the head.

Neuralgia of the nerves of the head and neck, backache, tremor of the limbs, "a giving way at the knees," or partial, or total but temporary, powerlessness of the arms or legs are frequently met with.

Any of these symptoms and signs may appear in varying degree; and when the "change" is over, all these complaints may gradually cease and the patient revert to her normal mental and physical condition. *Psychotherapy* can do more for the troubles of the climacterium than any other treatment.

CHAPTER XI

DRINKING AMONG WOMEN

THE CURE OF INEBRIETY

STATISTICS of drunkenness among women appear to prove that it is increasing rapidly.

Women, if they drink at all, should only drink when at table with their husbands or friends, and never at any other time. That rule alone will save them from all danger of forming a perilous habit. It would be better for every woman who wishes to remain sound and have sound offspring, and, still more for every woman who has any sort of nervous trouble, to be as nearly as possible an abstainer.

The predisposition that renders certain persons specially liable to become victims of alcoholism is of a twofold nature; it may consist of an attraction towards alcohol, in consequence of which the habit is very quickly established, or of an intolerance of alcohol, in consequence of which small quantities serve to produce brain disturbances.

The attraction towards alcohol is very often acquired. As the result of serious illness and exhausting diseases, persons previously abstainers, or only moderate drinkers, may develop a strong liking for it.

The tolerance of alcohol varies very greatly in different individuals. Some women are intoxicated by very small quantities. This intolerance is greatest in women who are predisposed to diseases of the nervous system, or whose nervous system is actually disordered, and those who exhibit mental instability. Such women, when once accustomed to alcohol, often experience an increasing sense of ill-being when deprived of it for any length of time, and their craving becomes uncontrollable.

Among the contributory causes are early training and example, grief, worry, jealousy, loneliness, ennui from lack of occupation, mental depression, and free access to alcohol. They take it for its power of lessening the feeling of fatigue and physical discomfort, and for the cheerfulness it inspires which makes the person forget her troubles.

Drunkenness is commonest in those who drink for oblivion or stupefaction, less in those who drink for stimulation and excitement. The woman who takes to drink in order to forget her misfortunes must be already a weak character, for to attain her end she must use increasing quantities of alcohol. Indulgence gives her temporary relief; the experiment is repeated; the power of the will is still further sapped; the consciousness of the practice, the sense of degradation, is now added to the pre-existing misery; and the remnants of self-restraint and of self-respect are swept away in the current of a resistless stream. The patient does not seek the pleasing sensations of intoxication, she drinks rather to escape from a state of sobriety which has become intolerable; it is the positive bliss of oblivion that she seeks eagerly and persistently. Resolutions to break herself of the habit may be made, but the patient has lost the capacity to maintain a resolution.

Those who drink for stimulation are usually steady drinkers. Before they can attempt any mental and physical task, they must have recourse to alcoholic stimulation. In them, a considerable quantity is required before intoxication is produced.

Most of the women I have had to treat had no taste for alcohol, but once they were given a glass to drink the craving was induced and they could no longer stop themselves. In such women there is a recurrent drink mania; and between the attacks, there is no strong desire for alcohol, and many women actually dislike it. They are conscious of their condition, which they deplore, and recognise their impotence to mend. They constantly oscillate between the desire to satisfy their craving and the sincere desire to resist, because they are conscious of the dreadful consequences of their intemperance. Their striving to resist explains why their excesses occur periodically in a recurrent manner. They are the victims of occasion, and would never become drunkards if it were possible for them to live always under tutelage. After the excess is over, the patient is full of repentance, asks for forgiveness and vows never to do it again; but unless treated, all their good resolutions vanish at the first opportunity.

Other women, again, who have acquired the taste for alcohol and yet are thoroughly ashamed of their bad habits, drink secretly; and until the habit becomes established, when certain symptoms appear which betray the chronic alcoholic, the husband and friends may remain ignorant of the evil tendency. So insidiously does the habit commence and grow, so secretly is it practised and the habit formed, that it is some time before the dreadful knowledge forces itself upon the friends. Their tears and solicitations, and the most vigilant watching, are as naught to the victim who has entered once into the meshes of this passion for the best of all possible reasons—that the power of the patient to keep the promise of reform is *nil*.

Often there is nothing to show in the " secret " drinker but persistent gastric derangement. As a rule, the appetite returns and the patient recovers her digestive powers very soon after the alcohol habit is given up.

Others suffer from such acute pains in their limbs—alcoholic neuritis—that they must seek relief and thus the habit is discovered.

Among other symptoms from which the female drunkard is apt to suffer are tremors, restlessness, insomnia, and delirium tremens. This last occurs chiefly in the type of women who come before the police courts as " drunk and disorderly " ; the other symptoms occur in the chronic secret drinker.

In women drunkenness and immorality often go together. Even when there is no intellectual decay, there is a deterioration in the moral sphere. Cunning and untruthfulness are leading characteristics of the dipsomaniac. Persons who, up to the time of their contracting the disease, were regarded as uniformly truthful and honest in every relation of life, now totally disregard the good opinion of their friends. There is no strategy, no humiliation, no sacrifice too great for the purpose of obtaining the, to them, necessary stimulant.

The drinking habit is confined to no one class of women. In fact, the women I have had to treat have all been women of culture and refinement. Often the habit has its origin in physical conditions which are more or less amenable to treatment. It will not do for us to attribute in all cases to mental depravity, or to blameworthy avoidance of mental effort, what is little, if at all, under the patient's control. The cure will depend in large measure on a correct diagnosis of the physical condition, and an intelligent comprehension of the individuality of the patient.

It has been freely stated that when a woman becomes an inebriate she may be regarded as hopeless; in fact, that her reformation is practically impossible. Such expressions of opinion are entirely erroneous, and do harm by instilling into the minds of inebriate women the hopelessness of struggling against their failing. I have had a large number of inebriate women in private care, secret drinkers as well as women whose vocation exposes them to the temptation of drink; and can vouch that quite a number of them have become teetotallers and remained such. If a patient is willing to be treated, there is as a rule no difficulty in curing her. Only the women without sober intervals, and who have already lost all sense of shame and responsibility, are difficult to treat in private care. For these the only hope is the "inebriate home."

Those patients who honestly desire to correct the habit, but merely lack the power, make good subjects for treatment. There are many patients who suffer from dipsomania at irregular intervals who recognise their danger and sincerely wish to be cured. When they regain normal consciousness, they experience a feeling of profound despair and make the most solemn promises, perhaps actually drinking nothing but water; but in a few weeks or months the whole affair begins again. These are the cases in which *treatment by suggestion* is most successful. The result has, in many cases, been remarkable. They are not put to sleep, but merely in a passive state of somnolence, in which all their muscles are relaxed; they breathe deeply and regularly, and their mind is focussed exclusively on the subject of advice. Having acquainted myself beforehand with the patient's dominant thoughts, beliefs, and mental environment, and, above all, having secured her confidence, I talk sympathetically to her in regard to her failing, impressing upon her that she will no longer be a slave of the vice which is wrecking her life. She is told that alcohol in any form will disgust her, that she will have such a horror of the moral degradation to which alcohol leads that she will find it quite easy to abstain. Appeal is made to her better feelings. Former ideals, loves, and affections, now slumbering, are roused, so that her future appears bright to her and her depression is overcome. The best instincts have to be discovered and engaged. There is some element of good in every human being, and this must be elicited and drawn out.

I also try to picture before her mind the awful appearance of herself when intoxicated, the disgust with which her husband and her children, or anyone else whom she respects or holds dear, observes her; and I tell her that when she feels tempted, this picture will be so vivid before her eyes that she will experience no difficulty whatever in withstanding the temptation.

Of course, one must in all cases try to discover the physical or moral conditions that determine the habit; and must treat the exhaustion or cause of the exhaustion by hygienic and other means. Any suggestion that is made must be in harmony with the natural feelings of the patient, so that she realises it is her own strength of will, and not the physician's influence, which is curing her of her habits.

Individuality by this method is not destroyed nor weakened, but, on the contrary, greatly strengthened. Self-control is not diminished, but the reverse; the subject is made able to do the thing which in her best moments she desired to do, but was not able to accomplish unaided.

What has been said of the drink habit is equally true of the DRUG HABIT and other pernicious habits. The danger of forming a habit is great with normal persons, but is still greater when drugs are in the hands of careless or neurotic persons. The treatment of the drug habit is similar to that of the drink habit. Treatment by "suggestion" offers, in my experience, the best chance of cure.

CHAPTER XII

PHYSICAL METHODS OF TREATMENT

In the treatment of functional nervous disorders, we must not ignore the physical needs of the patient. We must raise the vital energy and nervous force of the patient before we apply psychic treatment. Often the nervous system is so exhausted that the patient has no will-power left, lacks the necessary energy to carry out her good intentions. Even in functional affections, there is some nutritional or other disturbance, some change in the biochemistry of the tissues, so that it is not sufficient to restore the mental condition; we must also restore the health of the organisation with which mind is connected, and upon the normal state of which its soundness depends.

The first thing to do is to put the patient on the best physical basis, then we have solved part of the problem in regard to the mental condition. Even if there be no actual disease anywhere about the body, the patient, owing to her habitual indulgence of morbid thoughts or habits, has weakened her constitution ; and may suffer from a state of nervous exhaustion or irritability which requires our treatment on established lines.

The object of " Christian Science " and similar cults is " to destroy the patient's belief in her physical condition," and that is where the harm arises ; for the physical state must be treated as well as the mental attitude of the patient, otherwise no cure, or at least no permanent cure, is possible. We do not deny that many of these cults have effected cures ; but the cures they may have produced are such as could have been brought about by any conscientious physician acquainted with modern psychotherapy. Whatever ills of humanity it is possible by any means to relieve, legitimate medicine is able to cope with. Medical men may have neglected the mental side of disease too long, but psychotherapeutics is now rapidly spreading ; and there is no need for any patient nowadays, whether suffering from physical, mental, or moral defects, to seek the aid of persons unqualified in the science of medicine.

When we have raised the vital energy, the local symptoms often disappear. But the patient too frequently makes this mistake, that she ignores her general condition, and seeks aid for her particular local ailment, by following the lines of some advertised remedy or method of treatment. No qualified physician would be led away by the patient to treat individual symptoms and to prescribe specially for headaches, backaches, pains in the limbs, dyspepsia, palpitation, insomnia, and the rest. Indeed, a too careful attention to local symptoms in the nervous patient is often distinctly injurious, and tends to foster in her mind the belief that she is physically ill, of which it should be the chief object of treatment to disabuse her mind. Thus, if too much care is devoted to physical examination, the patient is liable to think that, after all, there must be something organically wrong for the doctor to take such time and trouble. Frequently these patients have already been examined by well-known experts, whose report may be available, so that a quick confirmatory examination may be all that is necessary. It is not hereby implied that the physical examination should be neglected, only that care should be taken not to rouse unduly the patient's fears.

Do what we will, every patient expects a prescription. The popular belief in the all-embracing efficacy of DRUGS is widespread. The advance of civilisation has done little or nothing to decrease the hopeful spirit which throughout the ages has prompted mankind to believe in the curative power of drugs. No doubt the cut-and-dry method of prescribing in the out-patient departments of hospitals, where there is no time for studying the individuality of the patient, is responsible to some extent for the implicit belief in the physic bottle. The patient wishes for immediate relief and cure; she believes that the physician who has studied so much has some remedy already prepared for such disease, and that what she will have to do is to go to the pharmacist and get it. She listens only distractedly to the counsels of hygiene which the serious physician gives her, and she looks upon them merely as measures intended to favour the medicinal action, which no doubt they often are.

Most patients, educated as well as uneducated, still believe that there has been no treatment unless a medicine is prescribed. It is very disappointing when, after we have been giving advice for about an hour and flattering ourselves on having made an impression, we are met with the question on leaving: "Are you not going to give me a prescription?" The aristocratic patient no more believes that her disorder can be cured without the aid of a prescription than her poorer fellow-mortal who, when ill, attends regularly at the hospital or dispensary in order to obtain the bottle of physic which she looks upon as indispensable to the restoration of her health.

The sole idea of treatment amongst the public seems to be that certain preparations relieve certain symptoms, and that when particular phenomena present themselves the same remedies must be used, no matter what the origin of these symptoms. Taking drugs without consultation with a medicinal practitioner is undoubtedly on the increase, and it is the delight of some individuals to advise their friends to take certain things for the relief of their ills. Many of the popular preparations are, of course, harmless, only containing simple ingredients; but when more potent remedies are used—for example, narcotics—the risk becomes formidable.

It is seldom that a month passes without there being recorded in considerable detail cases in which people, who have habitually dosed their systems with excessive quantities of narcotic drugs, overstep the limit which in safety, to life at least, is possible, and perish miserably as a result of their indiscretions. But death is not the worst sequel for the drug-taker in many cases. Indeed, it is for her a rest from her grievous troubles. But there is much to be endured before that consummation is reached. There is the steady diminution of resisting power, the physical deterioration, the cry of the tissues for more and more of the stimulant, and in many cases a gradual moral degradation. It is, of course, true that in many cases the taking of drugs is but a symptom of an unstable nervous organisation. Apparently a habit may be formed in regard to any drug, no matter how nauseous and unpalatable it may be; a certain effect is obtained, and this seems to be sufficient to atone for other effects which are unpleasant and noxious.

We have sometimes to recommend ISOLATION in a nursing home, but isolation is necessary only in those cases where the friends or relatives do not exercise a wholesome influence on the patient; or where they are impatient with the invalid, or else where they are the opposite, too loving and indulgent, so that the patient makes no effort to rouse herself.

The isolation cure implies rest in bed, but we must remember that while most patients are only too glad to stay in bed, others are rendered so irritable and restless by it that the term "rest in bed" becomes wholly a misnomer.

DIETING, combined with rest, is excellent,

especially when there is severe nervous exhaustion and we require to raise the constitutional strength of the patient. The employment of methodical overfeeding proves useful in conditions of malnutrition, and is due to the recognition of the possibility of excessive quantities of food being assimilated, in spite of diminished functional capacity of the alimentary organs. The object aimed at is the administration of a large amount of highly nutritious food in a relatively small volume at short intervals, the quantity being gradually increased to two or three times the customary amount.

The converse of overfeeding is underfeeding. This is recommended by numerous physicians who are advocates of vegetarian diet. Such reduction cure must be continuous, as no permanent good can follow a course of four or six weeks if the patient reverts to her former habits.

While rest cure is of use in some cases, others are better helped by the WORK CURE, the work chosen being one in which the patient takes pleasure. It must not be too severe or too long continued.

Many women are far too much indoors and a CHANGE OF SCENE, besides giving relief from household duties and family worries, is to be recommended on account of the change of air and environment. Sunshine contributes to physical energy and mental cheer. Physical exercise is to be recommended at the same time as change of scene. It greatly aids in the burning up of bodily poisons; and thus relieves the mind from the depression which results from the accumulation of the toxic substances in the blood stream. However, if we recommend any form of exercise to such patients, it often is the case that they lack the persistency to persevere with it. Exercise for the mere sake of exercise is so uninteresting a procedure that few women will follow it out. An element of interest must be introduced, and this is furnished by the various "sports" which are now open for both men and women.

The great aim in the treatment of nervous disorders should be to raise the vitality and the tone of the nervous system of the patient, besides the application of psychotherapy. There is a difference in vital energy. One person has more of it than another; one recovers rapidly and surely after a nervous breakdown, while another drags along through years of semi-invalidism. Functional nervous disorder is due to an enfeeblement of nerve force, and to this the treatment must be directed as well as to the mental symptoms. Now, a valuable instrument for raising the tone of the nervous system, the resisting power and general vitality of the patient, is electricity.

ELECTRICITY for the treatment of nervous disorders is still not used as extensively as it might be. There are several reasons for this neglect. One is, that until recently there was a great lack of precision in the knowledge possessed concerning it. Besides this, electricity is an agent which, in its manifestations, has always appealed to the human imagination. It has been credited with marvellous powers of cure, and, in the hands of the unscrupulous quack, has been utilised to impress that large section of the public which is gullible ; but with the effect on the medical mind of raising distrust of and prejudice against a therapeutic measure for which marvellous powers were claimed. Lay practitioners may understand the machine they are using, but they know little or nothing of the anatomy and physiology and the diseases of the nervous system. Even if the electricity is applied in accordance with the instructions received from a medical man, there is the mental element in all nervous disorders, which must never be neglected, and none but a qualified physician can be a skilled psychotherapist. The consequences of electrical applications in the hands of non-medical persons may be disastrous. What can we expect when a man or woman, who has taken a three months' course in some hospital or quack medical institution, can set up in practice for himself or herself and advertise electrical treatment, in competition with men who spent five or six years on their medical education, and several years more on getting skilled in their specialty? Gradually the utilisation of electricity is passing out of the hands of pretenders and showmen, and its value and merit are becoming recognised by thoughtful men and scientific workers, who see in it a vast power for good if kept within the compass of its applicability. At one time physicians were uncertain as to the mode of action of electricity on the body; but during recent years medical electricity has been undergoing very important developments, to an extent scarcely realised by those who are not intimately associated with the subject. It is now much more scientifically understood, and electrical applications are correspondingly more accurate and reliable.

Often the nervous system is too exhausted for the patient to appreciate any psychotherapeutic influence. When by electrical, medicinal, or other treatment we have improved her general condition, she feels "fit" again, and her morbid fears or other abnormal feelings disappear without any special effort. On the other hand, where they are more deeply rooted, the patient's attendances for electrical treatment give us an opportunity—which we might not get otherwise—of employing such "suggestion" therapy, persuasive and analytical methods, as may suit her individuality; and thus both her mental and physical health are restored.

CHAPTER XIII

GENERAL PSYCHOTHERAPY

MORAL ADVICE AND PERSUASION

THE physician practising psychotherapy should not only be a practical psychologist who can see, so to say, through the patient, but he ought to be, before all, a man of heart who knows how to put himself in the place of those who suffer. The patient should immediately feel that the physician is a friend with no idea but to cure her. All psychotherapy presupposes the existence of a special sort of sensibility in the physician; but it is a fact that the manner in which the patient acts towards the physician is quite as important a factor in successful psychic treatment as is the demeanour of the physician himself. It is this psychic contact which plays the determining rôle in psychotherapy. Without it, medicines may be administered, and surgical operations performed effectively, but successful suggestions cannot be implanted.

The application of psychotherapy demands a great deal of time and patience. It is this fact which makes its practice impossible for many physicians. At the outset, many of these nervous patients think it necessary to furnish all sorts of details of their life history, a great many having no bearing on their complaint. They frequently relate events in the most circumscribed manner, treating trivial details as if they were of the greatest importance, not forgetting for instance when giving a date, the state of the weather on that day, whom they met at the time, and so on. The more considerate of this class of patients send one their history by post, writing all they wish to say. This is certainly much appreciated by the busy doctor, though the report is sometimes twenty to thirty pages long and illegibly written. The physician who would try to hurry his patient or receive her complaints restlessly, or without interest, or worse still, with a hint that they are foolish or imaginary, would never be successful in this method of treatment. Formerly these patients were told there was nothing the matter with them; but nowadays we know, however exaggerated their complaints may be, the exaggeration is not simulation, and that the patients actually suffer even if the existence of any disorder cannot be demonstrated objectively.

Often the patient imagines her illness to be serious, and the idea is then difficult to dislodge. In such a case all depends on the confidence the patient has in the physician and his skill. If the patient lacks confidence in the physician, she fails to carry out his instructions with that accuracy and exactness of detail which is at all times the secret of success. Many a patient becomes chronic, when she might have been cured long ago, simply because she does not follow out the physician's instructions; but allows herself to be easily persuaded by her too anxious friends to consult this man or that man, or to take this or that quack medicine, which cured Mrs. So-and-so when everybody had given her up. It is extraordinary the numbers of people these patients consult, and I need scarcely say that the result is very unfortunate for the patient.

There must be no timidity or therapeutic indecision on the part of the doctor. A nervous patient only gets better when she believes that she is going to get better; and therefore the physician does not succeed in his work, except when he has a confident expectation of the success of his treatment. Though the nervous patient may complain of loss of memory in other respects, she is usually endowed with an excellent memory for everything that pertains to her condition and her health; and, paying great attention to the words of her physician, she will seize upon the slightest indication that can give her hope or otherwise.

It is not alone by an appeal to the understanding that we should try to succeed, but also by the introduction of an emotional element which will cheer the patient. Her point of view, her attitude of mind, beliefs, and habits of thought, may have to be modified not only by the introduction of new points of view, and of data drawn from the wider experience of the physician, by the instruction in the meaning of symptoms, and of duties to be assumed but too long neglected, but also by the suggestion of expectations that justly may be fulfilled, of ambitions that can rightfully be entertained, and of confidence, hope, and the joy of a brighter outlook of life. The physician who builds up a new confidence in a happy future most easily brings to the patient that self-control and energy which is the greatest of helping agencies. To be successful, therefore, the physician must know exactly what chords to strike that are likely to respond, and for this purpose a knowledge of the patient's character, outer and inner history, is an essential preliminary.

We must first of all eliminate any organic sources of irritation; then we may examine the habits of the patient for the source of the trouble. Often some departure from hygienic living, either physical or mental, will be found to be the starting-point. This may have been unavoidable when it occurred, or have been thought so, or what is more likely, not thought about at all until the mischief was done. We may have to insist on the changing of bad habits and the formation of good habits. Unfortunately, most patients do not want to change their habits. They come to the doctor to obtain some remedy, generally medicine, that will, without further inconvenience to themselves, rid them of certain discomforting symptoms; and they resent interference with their accustomed ways.

Often the cause of the nervous trouble lies in the unsystematic, disorderly habit of the patient as regards her daily duties, which in consequence have become a source of worry and fatigue. Such a patient should make as many as possible of the things she has to do automatic by repetition. For example, mere punctuality and system in the matter of doing minor things, let us say, her household duties, would relieve her of one form of worry, save her many small anxieties; and so do away with the constant making of decisions and the over-consideration of trifles. By advising system for the economising of time and energy, I do not mean to recommend that sort of craze for orderliness which so often defeats itself, and causes more trouble than it brings help. It is possible to make a veritable obsession of tidiness and order. System is wanted, a methodical, planned system, elastic enough to be adaptable, and yet exact enough to hold one to the performance of certain duties at certain stated times. Hours for rest, hours for leisure, hours for pleasure, must enter into such a schedule, as well as definite time for work and food and duty. The patient should rise daily at the same hour, have her meals punctually; and when she goes out, she should go with a list of what she intends to do in the order in which she means to do it. Then she will not need to worry at having forgotten something and have to go over the same ground again. Such advice about the management of life in minor matters is needed, because it cannot be too often repeated that it is the little troubles of life that cause the most breakdowns, not the great hurts or efforts. A hundred small anxieties or worries are like so much sand in the axles, and are far more dangerous and damaging than is the one big stone which the wheels bump over somehow, roughly perhaps, but successfully.

Another common cause of nervous trouble is insufficient rest, by which I mean not merely physical quiet but also mental peace. A practice to be recommended in such cases, and one, indeed, that is of benefit to most nervous patients of whatever sort, is that of physical and mental relaxation daily at a fixed time. How best to seek such rest is a matter depending on the conditions of the person and her environment. When the body and mind are tranquil, the thoughts and emotions are normally and healthfully formed and the brain centres are able to carry on their work with the expenditure of a minimum amount of energy.

Sometimes the fundamental difficulty is a sort of derangement of moral perspective. Trifles have come to occupy the foreground so completely that they obscure or altogether hide the larger and more important things of life. This is often because trifles do really and unavoidably occupy too large a share of the patient's daily attention. Generally speaking, the mental life of many women is worried out of them in the slavery of petty housework and childish vanities, deadening in themselves and bound up with all sorts of cares and vexations. In view of this, it is extremely necessary that a woman's horizon should be broadened, so that she can free herself from continually attaching too much importance to every little detail and thereby neglecting what is higher and more important.

Others have neither domestic nor other duties, indeed nothing that would distract them from perpetual self-contemplation and complaints that they are misunderstood. These women fail to adapt themselves to their environment, and frequently they poison their existence by perpetual lamentations. They complain of everyone and everything, and their grievances are without number. Very often they possess everything to make them happy, and yet they are never satisfied; the slightest cloud suffices to hide from them the sun, and trifles that another would not perceive affect their temper. Often their lamentations are merely the expression of wounded vanity and self-love, and are falsely regarded as due to their "nerves"; whereas it is the lack of self-control, in the first instance, that caused their nerves to get disordered.

Again, other women require to be warned

against useless social prejudices, above all against luxury, vanities, frivolous amusement, and especially against inordinate longing for enjoyment, which ruins normal pleasures and induces dissatisfaction and unhappiness from satiety.

In our search for mental causes, we must be as conscientious as we are accustomed to be in our physical investigations. We must search the mind of the patient for the source of her discomfort in exactly the same spirit as we search the body for physical discomfort. We shall generally find some unhealthy mental states, such as depressing emotions, apprehensions and fears, illogical doubts and scruples, habits of morbid introspection and self-consciousness, excessive concentration of the attention on particular organs, and so on. Some patients require to be counselled to suppress extravagant feelings, to discourage undue expression of emotions of all kinds, to meet worries tranquilly, make decisions without over-consideration; and to remember that although one must to some extent examine oneself to do these things successfully, one must not get too much wrapped up in one's symptoms.

Many nervous patients reason inconsistently, or their reason works in the wrong direction.

Even when they reason quite correctly, it is often from false premises. For example, many a patient falsely believes that deprivation of sleep is a direct sign of both physical and mental breakdown; assuming this statement to be correct, she gets into a state of extreme anxiety when for any reason her sleep is interfered with. The result of this anxiety very naturally is such a fixation of the attention upon her physical and mental condition that sleep for this very reason becomes increasingly difficult. Thus a vicious circle is formed. The treatment of this situation is in the first place to explain to the patient that she has a wrong conception of the significance of sleep; that complete physical and mental rest without sleep would suffice to restore her for the work of the succeeding day; and finally that if she would compose herself to such complete physical and mental rest, sleep would naturally follow.

Not infrequently there is no control over the imagination. The imagination is one of the most useful powers of the mind, when normally exercised; but it is also often engaged in creating mischief, fictitious difficulties, and even false diseases and unreal disorders of the body. It is self-evident, therefore, that such persons need to have their current of imagination arrested, or turned from a diseased into a healthy channel. By getting a patient interested outside of herself, we prevent her from struggling with her preoccupations, and from feeling any apprehension or fear concerning her obsessions; and they, no longer arousing any feeling, lose their significance, and the patient forgets them.

From what has been said it should have become already evident to the reader:

1. That in psychotherapy we treat the patient and not alone the disease;

2. That psychotherapy is not mere "faith healing"; and

3. That its most successful employment is in association with moral hygiene and moral orthopædics.

CHAPTER XIV

THE SUBCONSCIOUS MIND

PSYCHO-ANALYTIC TREATMENT OF NERVOUS DISORDERS

It is well known that the bodily functions can be influenced by our mental acts, and that certain states of mind are apt to be accompanied by various derangements of the functions of the body. Everyone knows how the receipt of an unpleasant letter may make us lose all appetite for food, and even cause us indigestion or headache, how fear may actually paralyse the muscles and keep us "rooted to the spot," how sudden shock will sometimes result in instant death, how long-continued grief or mental strain will sap the strength of the body. And it is no less a fact of mental observation that when healthy mental states are substituted for unhealthy ones, the functional derangements of the body tend to disappear.

On the other hand, it is owing to the same organisation that our mental dispositions can be influenced by the bodily functions. Nobody is constantly the same self. Not only is one a different self at different periods of one's life and in different circumstances, but also on different days, according to one's bodily states: sanguine and optimistic, gloomy and pessimistic, frank and genial, reserved and suspicious, apathetic or energetic. Although our intellectual powers remain the same, our judgment of the objective world and our relations to it are quite changed, because of the change in our moods and the bodily states which they imply.

Without giving any further illustrations, it will be admitted that there is ample evidence of the interaction between mind and body, that the body can be weakened through the agency of the mind and strengthened also by the same agency.

We are not conscious of the various functions of the organic life of the body, which go on in quiet harmony, with the nicest adaptations of means to an end throughout its complex mechanism. We are not conscious of the working of these processes; we are conscious only of the results and know nothing of the existence of the machinery, unless it becomes disturbed in one or other of its functions, and the message it then sends to the brain is felt as a discomfort or " pain." Nor are we conscious of our feelings until they have actually appeared. All our feelings—love, fear, anger, etc.—arise spontaneously without our knowledge. We can control them only after we have become conscious of them. As a rule, it is only the result of a mental event that we are conscious of, the actual origin and working remains obscure.

Even in the cleverest of us, in the ordinary mental operations of our daily life, there is not so much consciousness as is commonly assumed. A sensation, thought, or motion requires to be of a certain magnitude or intensity, and to persist before the mind for a certain time, to make us conscious of it. An act of attention, that is, an act of concentration—by which we mean the fixing of the mind intently upon one particular object to the exclusion for the time of all other objects that solicit its notice—is necessary to every exertion of consciousness. Without some degree of attention no impression of any duration can be made on the mind, or retained by the memory. The more consciousness is concentrated upon any new operation, the more readily it is mastered and impressed upon the memory; but as we acquire facility and skill in the operation, and the memory acquires strength, we become less conscious. The more we cultivate and train any power or faculty, the more easily and rapidly does it perform its work, the less is consciousness concerned in it, and the less does it suffer from fatigue.

Acts, which are at first executed slowly and with full consciousness and attention, become gradually less and less perceptible as they gain in ease and rapidity by repetition, till they fall below the minimum necessary for consciousness, and become unconscious, or rather subconscious. In our first attempts to walk, to write, to play on an instrument, or to carry on any other operation, we are intensely conscious of every movement that we make. By degrees, as we acquire more ease and dexterity in their performance, we become less and less conscious of them, till we may come to perform them quite unconsciously. Did everything that exists in the mind exist there consciously, or did every time that an idea occurred to the mind all the other ideas that had at any time been associated with it come along with it, and a selection have to be consciously made of the right one, inconvenience and loss of time could not fail to result. In some persons, from habit or lack of proper training, an idea in the mind immediately recalls a number of other ideas, having more or less, and sometimes very little, connection with it—thus distracting the mind with a multitude of thoughts, making the selection of the best a conscious act, producing hesitation and indecision, and causing loss of time.

The more we concentrate our attention on a particular subject, the less we notice other concurrent impressions. For example, in listening to a conversation we receive impressions not only of the words uttered, but also of the sounds in the air, and of its temperature, of odours, the forms, colours, lights and shades—all associating themselves with the thoughts conveyed—but we exclude all these impressions from our consciousness, although they may be noticed by our subconsciousness.

The more we concentrate on a subject in hand, the less we notice also our internal sensations; so that in times of real danger the body may feel no pain, no matter how severe the injury. Even a coward often acts under circumstances of unavoidable danger with the same coolness, and evinces the same presence of mind, as the bravest man. The most timid woman, under such circumstances, will fight like a demon, and display preternatural strength and courage for the perservation of her own life, or that of her offspring.

All our latent memories are stored in our

subconscious mind. Not a millionth part of the mental possessions exist in our consciousness at any one time. We may forget objects and events —that is to say, we may dismiss them from our consciousness, but they are stored up in our subconsciousness to the end of our days. We may be able to call them into consciousness when we wish to do so, but at other times the mind is unconscious of their existence. There are a multitude of events which are so completely forgotten that no effort of the will can revive them, which may nevertheless be reproduced with intense vividness under certain physical conditions, as in the act of drowning or in a state of delirium.

It is not to be supposed, however, that these unconscious or subconscious impressions or thoughts exert no influence upon the mind. The brain being the instrument of the mind, every impression we receive, every thought we think, as well as every action we do, causes some change in that structure; and this change is permanent, forming an imperishable record of all that we have experienced, thought, or done in the past. These impressions, thoughts, and actions may never again come before our consciousness; yet they will remain in that vast subconscious or subliminal region of the mind, unconsciously moulding and fashioning our subsequent thoughts and actions. Every thought we have entertained, and every act we have done throughout our past life, make their influence felt in the way of building up our present knowledge, or in guiding our everyday actions. Many things of which we have no recollection that we have even noticed them, innumerable experiences which never attracted our attention, are stored up similarly, and may exercise an influence over us of which we are not conscious. Many minds are moody, morose, melancholy, excitable, irritable, immoral, unbalanced solely because of the overpowering influence of some memory of a past experience, which remains subconsciously in operation after conscious thought on the occurrence has ceased and the person has apparently forgotten the incident.

In normal everyday life, disagreeable or painful thoughts are always forgotten ; we intentionally or even unconsciously push them out of consciousness, so as to free ourselves from disagreeable feelings or pain. Sometimes, however, a disagreeable incident remains in our unconscious memory. Then, because we have no control over it, it cannot run its normal course and, therefore, becomes converted or changed into a pathological condition.

Repressed emotions are the mischief-makers at the bottom of many of the functional disorders, especially hysteria. If they are given an opportunity to complete themselves, if the patient in a state of relaxation and passivity is asked to talk out these painful experiences, to bring them vividly before her mind, they cease from troubling and a decided therapeutic effect is the result. The method of digging out this buried complex and bringing it to light or consciousness, and therefore to conscious control, is called *psycho-analysis*.

Nothing happens to us amiss; there is no such thing as non-significant experience. Every bit of experience, the seemingly most insignificant quite as much as the tragically significant, leaves its trace. In women it is often experiences and desires of the past which have been submerged in the mind by the current of later events, and have passed out of the present field of consciousness; but though submerged in this way they have not ceased to act upon the current above, and occasionally obtrude themselves in the shape of phenomena of which the patient complains. Some mental or emotional shock has occurred in the past life of the patient, and has become buried or forgotten in a state of subconsciousness, where it becomes the cause of the patient's present nervous symptoms; or some desire arising from a highly active instinct which for conventional or other reasons had to be suppressed, leaves a trail in the nervous centres which shows itself in disordered nervous function in later years. This experience or desire sinks, if one may so say, from the conscious to the subconscious region. Thus a conflict or disharmony is set up between the main stream of conscious personal life and the submerged or subconscious mental state. There is a lack of unity in the inner life, because this suppressed thought or emotion or wish is not at one with the personality as a whole.

Painful sensations are in the ordinary course of life usually "worked off." An insulted person relieves the feelings by strong language, grief is neutralised by tears, while in many other cases time may heal the wounded feelings. If, however, for any reason no relief is obtained, there is the possibility in certain cases of such painful experiences acting like foreign bodies in the brain; and though relegated to the subconscious part of the mind they are never destroyed, and are apt in certain circumstances to become active and to come into conflict with the conscious mind. Thus events which we have done our best to forget may crop up again. A woman, for example, in early adult life is subjected to the stress of a love-affair, accompanied by circumstances which her education has taught her to regard as discreditable, and in which social convention demands that she should hide the expression of her emotions. The stress over, she endeavours deliberately to erase the writing on that page of her memory which recorded it, and to a large extent she succeeds; but, nevertheless, the suppressed emotion, having missed the usual channels by which it ordinarily becomes declared, ferments, to use a very crude metaphor, and sooner or later shows itself in certain phenomena we associate with nervous disorders.

Psycho-analysis throws light upon the origin of habits and idiosyncrasies of all kinds and upon many obscure problems of everyday life. The instinctive dislikes, which so frequently influence conduct for no obvious cause, mannerisms and odd gestures, uncalled-for explosions of temper, inexplicable waves of sadness, sudden untimely merriment, blind unreasoning prejudices, are to be attributed to past experiences and old conflicts, which, though quite forgotten, may be discoverable by psycho-analysis. When disturbing factors that have been repressed or ignored are frankly faced, when the nature of the conflict is fully understood and the whole personality is summoned to take part in it, healthy influences have a chance of prevailing.

One method of treatment, therefore, is based upon the search for this subconscious painful memory, either through conversation with the patient or by the recital and the revival of forgotten scenes. I am not here advancing that it is always desirable to dig where such has been discreetly buried; but it remains nevertheless true that there are cases in which a resurrection of the past is the only method whereby we can hope for relief of present symptoms. By psycho-analysis, the skilled psychologist lays bare to the patient's view the concealed cause of her suffering, and thereby deprives the cause of its power to do harm. Sometimes this can be done by careful and sympathetic cross-examination. We all know the beneficial influence of a heart to heart talk with a wise and trusted friend. The suppressed emotions find here an outlet and we feel better. It is this idea which lies at the basis of the psycho-analytic method.

This psycho-analytic method of treatment requires some amount of time, for nothing can be done until the patient has attained proper emotional composure, has overcome any existing depression or confusion, and manifests the necessary interest in the interview ; even then she may unfold reminiscences of painful nature only piecemeal, so that a considerable number of interviews may be necessary before a complete recovery is established.

When we succeed in inspiring such confidence in the patient that she reveals to us these buried reminiscences which, we know, are the source of all her troubles, it is usually easy to make all her nervous symptoms disappear. To cite one example only :—

A young woman, age thirty, single, became very strange in her behaviour, showed great irritability, and became very jealous of her younger sisters. She could not be induced to go to public places. Her dread of public places, she confessed, was due to a feeling that every man she saw was molesting her though he did not speak or move. She could not account for her feeling until one day when again talking to her confidentially, I discovered the solution. Some twelve years before, on a voyage to Australia, she made the acquaintance of a passenger on board the steamer, who made love to her and whose affection she reciprocated. To him it was merely a little affair to pass the time ; and since their destinations were not anywhere near to one another, his good-bye on leaving the ship was a final one. To her the affair was not a mere incident. It affected her whole personality; she had never told anyone of her experience and for some years was quite a normal girl. It was only at the age of thirty, when her younger sisters began to attract more attention than herself, that she worried, became jealous, and got these peculiar feelings which upset her mental equilibrium. It was evident that the event was relegated to her subconscious life and that the man whom she adored years ago was still making love to her in her dreams and reveries; at least he did so in her imagination, and she liked to dwell on it. Then the picture faded, to be revived some years after not by one man making love to her, but by an unhinged imagination fancying that every man was making overtures to her. Once the event was brought again fully before her consciousness, it only required mental discipline and a reasonable attitude on her part to bring her back to her normal senses.

CHAPTER XV

TREATMENT OF NERVOUS DISORDERS BY "SUGGESTION"

WITH EXAMPLES

THE mind and will of the nervous patient are essentially weak and vacillating; hence arises the necessity for the controlling influence and guiding efforts of a will superior to her own. What the patient wants is disciplined treatment under someone who, whilst having plenty of sympathy, can mix it with firmness and authority, so as to check the ramifications of disordered feeling and make her realise how to help herself. The object of the treatment is to make the patient mistress of herself. Most people lack the power of mental discipline. Their mind is constantly "wandering." It is not, as some people suppose, that they have not got enough brain, but that they have not got enough power to keep in order such brains as they have. Instead of having their thoughts and feelings under their control, the thoughts and feelings spring up unawares and control them. The mental condition of hysteria, the morbid doubts and fears of nervous exhaustion, abnormal impulses, perverted habits, and many other troubles, are largely due to this lack of control over the powers which constitute mind and character. The appropriate treatment is by "suggestion."

By "suggestion" treatment we do not mean hypnotism. Sleep is not necessary, nor desirable, but simply a passive subjective condition. We can thereby produce rest in over-active parts of the brain, and can strengthen the volitional control which the patient exercises over her thoughts and feelings. By this process the patient does not lose consciousness; she knows what is taking place, though she may close her eyes and be in a condition of mental abstraction in which her mind is passive and receptive. Any suggestion made in this state is received by the patient in full consciousness; it does not escape from the control of her personality; and if she is a docile subject, convinced of the intellectual superiority of the physician, quite disposed in consequence to obey him, and vividly impressed by the method and by what she expects of it, it is easy to understand that she accepts and carries out the suggestion that has been given to her. But this suggestion is, on ultimate analysis, only a suggestion received in the waking state, facilitated perhaps by the belief of the invalid in the efficacy of this mode of treatment and by the ceremonial associated with it. This kind of "suggestion" treatment presents no dangers whatever.

When a patient is put in a comfortable position, breathes rhythmically, relaxes her muscles, and is shown how to concentrate so as to shut out distracting and exciting thoughts and prevent the mind from wandering, she will gradually get into that passive, subjective condition, which is so favourable for suggestion and auto-suggestion. We can then talk to the patient about her ailment with far greater success, make her forget her aches and pains, put away doubts and misgivings, and get her to control irrational thoughts and morbid cravings.

Any resolution that is come to by the subject in that state is likely to be carried into action. Thus a patient whose will has become so defective that she is unable to break herself of a certain deleterious habit, can determine in this state that she will no longer give way to it; she states to herself the reasons why she ought not to give way to it, why it would be positively disastrous to her to go on as she has done—and she will find, when the temptation occurs again, that she has all her reflections so vividly brought before her, that it is comparatively easy to resist it.

That there is anything injurious to the most delicate person in listening to good advice gently communicated while the mind is thus at peace, it is impossible to believe. The weakening of the will, the invasion or enfeeblement of personality, which writers who have never practised this art affirm so confidently, is a mere fiction of the imagination. In no single instance have I witnessed such a thing; but in scores of instances have I achieved the opposite, namely, the strengthening of the will to resist obsessions and to overcome morbid feelings and habits which have held victims in bondage for years, thus leading to the beginning of a new and happier life.

Treatment by suggestion is of immeasurable value in the cure of muscular tremors, chronic neuralgia, functional paralysis, nervous dyspepsia, chronic headache, nervous debility, mental depression, obsessions and imperative ideas, perverted habits, loss of will-power, somnambulism, and hysteria.

This form of treatment applied by trained

medical men is free from danger, sensationalism, and quackery, and is quite different to the notions many people have of it. Those who lack success in this treatment, have either not been trained for it, or they cannot judge the suitability and suggestibility of the patient for it, or cannot give the proper suggestions in the right manner.

In the first place, let me emphasise the importance of a correct diagnosis in each case. This does not mean merely determining the name of the disease; it means obtaining a complete grasp of the patient's mental, moral, and physical condition—why she is ill; what prevents her from getting well; what, if any, cause is still in operation? Indeed, I am realising more and more that the successful psychotherapist must be first of all a skilled physician with a wide experience of men and women in health and disease; for it is the diagnosis not of the disease but of the patient which is all-important.

Secondly, I wish to point out, that we must not ignore the physical needs of the patient, but recognise that psychical treatment alone is insufficient without physical measures; for even if there be no actual disease present, the habitual indulgence of morbid thoughts or habits has so weakened the constitution that it requires treatment on established lines. Medicinal, hygienic, dietetic, physical and moral measures have all to be employed, according to the individuality of the patient and the nature of the complaint. The patient who has been treated by psychotherapy alone is likely to have a relapse, because the constitutional condition which has given rise to the complaint has not been attended to—on the other hand, the patient who has received constitutional treatment only, whether by medicine or other physical measure, may be still subject to her psychical abnormalities, because no attempt has been made to cure her of her morbid mental habits.

I do not wish it to appear that every case of nervous disorder treated by suggestion is cured, nor do I suggest that every case of nervous disorder should receive this form of treatment. A large number of cases treated in orthodox fashion by drugs and other methods recover. But the psychotherapist is not usually consulted until ordinary methods have been given a fair trial, and it is well to remember that when all other methods fail there is still a possibility of effecting a cure.

As a proof of the usefulness of the suggestion treatment, and as there is still considerable ignorance as to the kind of cases that are benefited by such treatment, I append a few examples.

A Case of *Morbid Blushing, Self-consciousness, and Mental Confusion*:—

A young lady, twenty-four years of age, teacher by occupation, felt greatly embarrassed in her work through being afflicted with inordinate and excessive blushing. It occurred mostly when holding a class or speaking to her superiors, when an excessive flush came to her face so as to attract the attention of everyone near her. But the most distressing symptom was the mental confusion which accompanied it. She became dazed, her presence of mind entirely forsook her and she could command neither thought nor word. This, of course, often made her appear ridiculous and caused her intense mortification. After a fortnight's treatment by suggestion in the waking state very marked improvement took place—both as regards blushing and the power of self-control. From that time she practised auto-suggestion, and so successfully that there was no return of the trouble.

Case of *Nervous Exhaustion, Morbid Flushings, and Giddiness* :—

A lady, aged forty-five, consulted me for nervousness and irritability of temper. She had for years experienced considerable anxiety in her family affairs, to which she attributed her illness. She complained of a sensation of weight and pressure at the top of the head and in the temples, and of giddiness, chiefly on stooping and looking upwards. Her memory and power of application were very much impaired. Whenever anything unexpected or disagreeable occurred, she became flushed in the face, and had a sensation of tingling resembling slight electric shocks running down her hands. The patient had become very stout during the last few years, and her muscles were flabby. She complained of palpitations of the heart and shortness of breath in walking, more especially on going upstairs, but there was no disease of the heart or lungs. She rarely took active exercise ; it only seemed to make her worse. Besides suggestion, this lady received galvanic treatment to the spine and head with most satisfactory results. All the morbid symptoms gradually yielded, and in less than four weeks she was a happy active woman, and could attend to her duties and take exercise without experiencing the slightest discomfort.

Case of *Obsession and Fear of Insanity*:—

Another patient was haunted by a coarse word which she had seen scribbled on some fence. The word was ever on her tongue. It had become the one subject of her waking thoughts and her dreams, and she dreaded that she might lose self-control and utter the obscene expression before other people. She was tortured by the constant fear that she was going to be insane, and no direct appeal would convince her that her fear was groundless. She was, however, susceptible to suggestion treatment and readily lapsed into the somnolent state, when she was told emphatically that she would lose her obsession and her morbid fear, that she could not become insane, that she would find a pleasure in existence that she had not known before, and would recover completely.

Case of *Nervous Exhaustion, Insomnia, Want of Appetite, and Depression*:—

A married woman, forty-eight years old, was nervous ever since her change began two years before. She had a good deal of discomfort, complete loss of appetite, gloomy ideas, general demoralisation, insomnia. Often she did not sleep until daybreak. If she slept she had nightmare, and woke in the morning with headache and giddiness. Constant tremor agitated her limbs, to such an extent that she could hardly pour out a glass of water. This nervous condition resisted all the ordinary treatment. After a few visits for "suggestion" treatment, she no longer felt the slightest discomfort, no more tremor, slept well without any disturbance, her appetite better than ever, and her melancholy had disappeared.

Case of *Morbid Fears* :—

The patient, one day out walking, crossed an open field, in which there was a bull grazing. She got a fright, felt faint, the heart beat rapidly, she perspired freely, and trembled all over. She felt, to use her own expression, "as if the end of the world was coming." Since then she has been afraid of open places, of public squares, fields, and parks. If she went into an open space unaccompanied, after a few steps she would be attacked with trembling and giddiness, her sight became blurred, she perspired and was obliged to retrace her steps. She was a reasonable woman in all other respects and open to suggestion, so that when the groundlessness of her fears was pointed out to her repeatedly, she gradually gained confidence and courage.

Case of *Hysteria with Vomiting and Insomnia*:—

Patient, twenty years of age, had nervous symptoms from an early age. Her father died, and on the news of his death she had a nervous paroxysm which recurred subsequently about once a week. The attacks were preceded by a sensation as of a foreign body rising from the stomach into the throat and a constriction of the upper part of the chest. At times she had cramps of the stomach and vomited freely. Insomnia was constant. At a preliminary interview, the patient was encouraged to talk freely and at length on her experience, mental state and symptoms. She objected to direct suggestion treatment. A course of electricity was therefore proposed to strengthen her nerves and cure her nervous dyspepsia, and by means of indirect suggestion her mental state was attended to. The fits, vomiting, and insomnia, ceased within a few days and she made a perfect recovery.

Case of *Hysteria with Somnambulism*:—

Patient, a girl fourteen years of age, disappeared from her country home at frequent intervals, and was found miles away after a day or two, wandering in the woods and fields, by the police, who returned her to her parents. The patient had no recollection of her doings, though once she took a ticket to go a few stations by train. She was of a " dreaming " disposition, and it was noticed that before the attacks she used to talk to herself and loved the " open air." She underwent the suggestion treatment and recovered. She was kept under observation for some months to make sure of no relapse.

Case of *Sexual Morbidity*:—

A young girl, eighteen years of age, with family history of insanity, intellectually highly gifted but given to excitement, fanciful exaggeration, and prevarication, showed indecent tendencies since her tenth year, and had to be kept from the company of men and male servants. When thwarted in her designs she would break out in a fury of temper. On examination, there was hyperæsthesia and abnormal sensation of pain in left half of body. In female company, she was reserved, in male she had no sense of shame. Medicinal and hygienic measures were tried first, but they only invigorated her, and her perversity continued. Her mother was desirous I should try hypnotism. The patient made an excellent subject, and in the trance was put *en rapport* with her mother, and told she would confide everything to her, and do exactly as she wished her to do. Her mother then lectured her as to her tendencies and their possible consequences, and made her promise to do work for which she was greatly gifted, in order to divert her thoughts, to behave properly on all occasions, and to show obedience to her in every respect. Except that I sent the patient to sleep, I had nothing more to do with her. Her mother gained more and more control over her. The girl got perfectly well and was married two years later.

Case of *Religious Scruples* :—

A lady, always devoutly religious, age thirty-two, suffered for two years from delusions that she was " lost," that her soul was damned and that she alone was to blame for her misfortune. In addition, she heard blasphemous voices which drove her to despair. She was to be certified for an asylum by the doctor who had been attending her. The husband as a last resource desired to consult some expert in the treatment of mental disorders; and although no definite promise could be made as to her cure, with the approval of the doctor treatment by suggestion was arranged. The patient being much wasted, medicinal and hygienic measures were prescribed for her, while the psychical treatment continued. Gradually she grew stronger, the voices diminished in power, she behaved properly at home, but the anxiety as to the future of her soul still remained until I explained to her one day in the somnolent state, that she had been ill, that all the morbid ideas arose as the result of an exhausted if not diseased body, but the fact that she feared for herself, showed that she was pure in spirit, and since it was the spirit that goes to heaven, and not the body, she need feel no anxiety. This explanation had the desired effect, and after a few more visits she was herself again. I heard about twelve months later that she remained perfectly well.

Case of *Nervous Exhaustion and Insomnia* :—

A lady, aged fifty-two, had undergone considerable anxiety, was nervous, irritable, and sleepless. She either did not go to sleep at all on getting into bed, or if she dropped asleep from utter weariness, she woke up again in about half an hour, and lay restless during the remainder of the night. Besides this, she complained of weakness in the back, of a feeling of great exhaustion, total disinclination to any exertion, and to bodily exercise of any kind. She was easily excited and worried by little things, and extremely intolerant of noise, or of being asked any questions. She was often troubled with a sense of vague alarm, and distressing sensations in the head. She disliked her meals and generally suffered from flatulence. Suggestion treatment was applied, with the result that she slept already during the first night uninterruptedly for five hours. After three weeks' treatment the patient felt like another woman, being able to exert herself both mentally and bodily, enjoying her meals, and taking an active interest in the concerns of daily life.

Case of *Chronic Nervous Dyspepsia* :—

Lady, aged thirty-two, emaciated, extremely nervous, had been unable to take any solid food for nearly twelve months, and even latterly liquid food, such as milk, beef-tea, etc., could not be retained. She vomited twice a day. She had been under various specialists, who had made proper physical and chemical examinations; and as she got worse instead of better the last doctor consulted thought it a suitable case for "suggestion." She started treatment in the condition described above and weighed then five stones eight pounds. She was put into a somnolent state in which suggestions that she would remember could be made. She made slow but definite improvement. The vomiting became less frequent, and after a fortnight she could eat minced meat and retain it. After a month she could eat vegetables and farinaceous food, and meat cut in small slices. After six weeks she ate like any ordinary person and required no further treatment. She reported herself a few weeks later quite well. Her weight by that time had risen to seven stones and four pounds.

Case of *Nervous Troubles after an Accident* :—

Married lady, aged fifty-eight, had a taxi-cab accident, resulting in numerous cuts about her face. Shortly after the injury she became so "nervous" that the slightest noise startled her and produced trembling of the legs so that she could scarcely stand. At the same time, she suffered from great mental depression with dominant idea of absolute general inability. She could not walk to the corner of the street without entire failure of strength, could not read ten lines without feeling that the brain was "giving out." For the same reason she could not visit, nor go to any place of amusement. Her sleep was disturbed by attacks of palpitation, which would wake her up in terror and perspiration. Suggestion treatment restored the patient entirely. First of all the sleeplessness, then her general nervousness and despondency disappeared.

Case of *Neuralgia* :—

A lady, aged sixty-four, had for eight years suffered from neuralgia in the right side of the face, which had first come on after a nervous breakdown and under anxious circumstances. Since then the neuralgia left her only occasionally, and when she came under my care she was not free from attacks for a single day. Fits of pain came on after the slightest movements of the lips, chiefly during mastication, and in speaking, gaping, coughing, and sneezing. She was generally free from pain at night. The severity of the suffering, according to her statement, was such as to drive her nearly mad, and she had not known any enjoyment of life during the last eight years. Her general health was tolerably good. Digestion was good, but the patient was obliged to take her food minced very fine, because otherwise the act of mastication hurt her very much. She was also obliged to avoid anything hot, as this caused severe pain. It is unnecessary to mention the various remedies which had been used for the relief of the pain, as nothing seemed to have had the slightest beneficial effect. I applied radium ionisation, at the same time using psychotherapeutics. The next morning she was in high spirits, as she had been quite free from pain during the remainder of the day and had been able to masticate and eat her dinner without any trouble. She had had a good night, and it was only at breakfast that the pain had to some extent returned, although not nearly as bad as before. After a few visits the pain disappeared entirely and she has continued perfectly well since.

Case of *Nervous Pains and Loss of Power in Lower Limbs :—*

A lady, forty-six years old, who had spent months in nursing her sick husband, suffered subsequently from pains in her back and limbs and loss of power in her legs. She dragged herself about her room with difficulty, limping badly and clinging to the furniture. It was impossible for her to go up or down stairs alone. When in bed she could not turn or sit up without crying out with the pain. She could only lie down slowly. On examination, no organic cause could be found. Suggestions were made in the waking condition, that the pain was diminishing, that she could walk without limping, that everything was in good order. At the same time the painful areas were stroked gently, and after a quarter of an hour she was told decidedly that she could now get up and walk properly. This she did, the first day with hesitation, but each day better, and after a week she was well.

Case of *Rhythmical Arm Jerks* :—

Patient, a girl of eighteen, anæmic, suffered for four months from rhythmical adductive and abductive movements of the right arm. Various remedies had been tried, her arm had also been fixed for some weeks in plaster of Paris, but without avail. Even during sleep the arm was not quiet and sometimes woke her. After a dozen visits at gradually extending intervals the involuntary movement ceased entirely.

Case of *Rheumatic Pains* :—

A married lady, aged thirty-two, was sent to me by her local doctor. She had for the past four years suffered from severe neuritis in the right arm and shoulder, with this peculiarity, that she never was actually free from pain, but suffered constantly; at times, however, much more acutely than at others. The arm was almost useless to the patient, as she found that the pain became much worse when she attempted to do anything with it, so that she dreaded using it at all. Her general health was otherwise tolerably good, and no particular cause could be assigned for the occurrence of the neuralgia. She had used a variety of remedial measures, but all to no purpose, and the pain was getting worse instead of better. After a fortnight's galvanic treatment together with suggestion the pain entirely disappeared, and two years later I had the satisfaction of ascertaining that the patient had been free from it ever since.

Case of *Spinal Pains* :—

A young lady, aged twenty-two, very tall and of sallow complexion, came under my care. She had grown rapidly, especially between her seventeenth and nineteenth year, and had been ailing ever since to such an extent as to cause her parents much uneasiness. Being of an impulsive and highly-gifted nature, she would take a passionate interest in certain things, and devote many hours of hard work to mastering a subject which attracted her imagination; after which she would be completely exhausted and prostrated for days or weeks and be unable to do anything whatever. She suffered periodically from excruciating pains in the lower part of the spine, especially on making a sudden movement. She was almost entirely incapacitated from taking active exercise, partly from pain and partly by weakness. Her appetite was fanciful and her digestion weak. She received electrical in addition to suggestion treatment for a month, when she was able to take active exercise, had normal digestion, had become stouter, and could walk for miles without fatigue. The pains which she used to feel in the spine had entirely disappeared.

Case of *Inebriety* :—

A lady, aged thirty-seven, married, came under my care. She had, in consequence of anxiety, got into a state of complete nervous derangement. She was utterly incapable of any mental or bodily exertion until after she had taken two ounces of brandy in the morning, and she was in the habit of consuming about a pint of spirit every day. She hated the very sight and smell of brandy, but if she did not take it such horrible thoughts came into her head as to render life intolerable. Her judgment and intellect were not impaired, but she had not the slightest control over the dreadful ideas which constantly flitted across her brain if not under the influence of alcohol. Various treatments had been tried until her own medical practitioner sent her to me for suggestion treatment. Within a week from the commencement of the treatment the patient was able to discontinue the brandy, and she attended at intervals for three months, during which period she took no spirits whatever, although she could easily have procured some if she wanted to. Her moral courage, her outlook on life, her general mental and bodily health had all improved; and her doctor reported to me a year later that she kept perfectly well and was cured of her morbid tendency.

Cure of *Morphia Habit by Suggestion*:—

Patient, a lady, forty years of age, in consequence of severe spinal and visceral pains became addicted to the morphia habit. She had numerous injection scars on her arms and thighs. As in all such cases, morphia only gave her temporary relief; and as soon as the effect wore off she complained again of agonising pains and was intolerant even of the slightest touch to her skin. The morphia habit had also changed her character, the chief disposition now being excessive affection for her friends one day and extreme jealousy and hatred the next day, inventing all sorts of scandalous stories against them to justify the change in her disposition towards them. The patient made a good subject, was put into the passive state readily, and while half awake the suggestion, that the pain had gone, acted successfully. Within half an hour she fell asleep. In another half-hour she woke of her own accord and talked for about fifteen minutes, when the pains recommenced. She was again sent to sleep and the suggestion made that she would keep perfectly well for the rest of the day. Her own local doctor, who continued the treatment initiated by me, reported two months later her complete recovery. There were none of those usual grave symptoms of disturbance in the brain and nervous system after the withdrawal of the drug, which make it so difficult to break the opium habit by any other method.

Case of *Spasmodic Contraction of Muscles, Loss of Power in Lower Extremities, Pain, Insomnia, and Mental Depression* :—

" Suggestion " is a mysterious power of which we still know very little. To show what remarkable cures can be performed by it, let me quote as a final example an experience, an account of which was published in *The Medical Press*, January 3rd, 1912.

The patient, a girl, twenty-two years old, was sent to me on November 13th by her medical attendant. According to the history furnished by him the girl had had St. Vitus's Dance, with heart complications (endocarditis), since she was ten years of age. At fifteen years of age she had acute rheumatism and was in bed for some weeks. At nineteen she had an attack of appendicitis which recurred, until in May last year the appendix was removed. The year previously, May, 1909, she took to the use of a Bath chair, apparently owing to an inability to walk without having pains and being prostrated. The patient suffered besides from insomnia owing to night terrors, her screams rousing the people in adjoining rooms. Mentally she was in a very depressed condition and talked little, nor would she smile. She was still using her Bath chair when she was brought to me. Her personal appearance was that of an invalid in a very feeble state, her body almost rolled up and her head turned to the right shoulder, as if suffering from wry-neck.

On her first visit I merely tested the suggestibility of the patient, and reported to her doctor that I had no doubt that I should be able to benefit her. On her next visit, November 16th, I attempted to hypnotise her, and was partially successful, and considerable improvement followed. On November 24th she came again, and this time fell under my influence within a few minutes. She did not actually fall asleep, but she could not open her eyes and was unable to move her limbs. I suggested that all the muscles would resume their normal position, that she would be free from pain, sleep well at night undisturbed by dreams and visions, and would be cheerful and talk freely. On rousing the patient her outward appearance had completely changed. She held herself erect, seemed happy and well. What happened afterwards is best told by quoting her sister's letter to me, dated November 29th :—

"After leaving your house on Friday we walked along Oxford Street, through the lower departments of Selfridge's, on to Marble Arch, and across the Park to St. George's Hospital, where we took an omnibus for home ; that, for a girl who has scarcely walked a yard and has been wheeled about in a Bath chair since two years ago last May, is little less than a miracle. She is sleeping splendidly and naturally. All her terrible night fears have ceased to trouble her—and us, as her screams used to rouse us all at times. Her new cheery outlook on things in general would be almost laughable if we were not so intensely thankful. It seems almost impossible—a fortnight ago an apparently incurable invalid, again and again unconscious in her Bath chair in the streets, and now to-day, and every day since your treatment began, a normal, cheerful girl who is able to move about and speak, and whom it is a pleasure to be with."

On December 1st the patient called again, perfectly well, but she drew my attention to the fact that she had been suffering all along from constipation and absence of her monthly periods, and enquired whether I could cure also these complaints by the same method. When she was again in a somnolent state I suggested to the patient that on being roused her bowels would act, and after that every morning regularly, and she should have her period within twenty-four hours. The patient had a good motion directly she was awakened, and as regards subsequent events I can quote her sister's words, as per letter of December 3rd :—

"You scarcely need telling, I suppose, that once more your suggestions have taken wonderful effect in the case of my sister. Her bowels have acted naturally yesterday morning and this morning, and her period arrived yesterday afternoon. I cease to wonder at anything now! Her sleep, speech, cheerfulness, erect carriage, proper method of breathing, interest in life—all restored; freedom given from pains everywhere, dread of being again ill taken away, and now action of the bowels and period produced."

INDEX

P

PRINTED BY
WILLIAM BRENDON AND SON, LTD
PLYMOUTH, ENGLAND